We Wait for a Miracle

MUHAMMAD H. ZAMAN

We Wait for a Miracle

Health Care and the Forcibly Displaced

JOHNS HOPKINS UNIVERSITY PRESS

Baltimore

© 2023 Johns Hopkins University Press
All rights reserved. Published 2023
Printed in the United States of America on acid-free paper
9 8 7 6 5 4 3 2 1

Johns Hopkins University Press
2715 North Charles Street
Baltimore, Maryland 21218
www.press.jhu.edu

Cataloging-in-Publication Data is available from the Library of Congress.
A catalog record for this book is available from the British Library.

ISBN: 978-1-4214-4730-8 (hardcover)
ISBN: 978-1-4214-4731-5 (ebook)

Special discounts are available for bulk purchases of this book. For more information, please contact Special Sales at specialsales@jh.edu.

Contents

Contents

Characters and Locations

Names of the main characters have been changed at their request to protect their identity. The dates and locations, however, have not been changed.

Colombia: Bogotá

Rafael. A lawyer, originally from Lecheria, Venezuela, but based in Colombia since 2017. Works with migrants and the local Venezuelan community in Bogotá on issues of access to health care and social services.

Dr. Vargas. A Colombian physician based in Bogotá.

South Sudan: Juba and Malakan

Malakan is a small town about 70 kilometers from Juba and located close to Wonduruba.

Rev. Henry. A pastor and a health care worker, originally from Malakan and currently living in Juba.

Solomon. Henry's brother.

Dr. Julius. A prominent senior doctor in Juba who works both in the public sector and in private practice.

Dr. James. An eye specialist originally from South Sudan but currently living in Zimbabwe.

Uganda: Bidi Bidi

One of the largest refugee camps in the world is located in Bidi Bidi, with a significant number of South Sudanese refugees living there. Solomon, Henry's brother, lived in the camps for several years; it is approximately 200 kilometers from Malakan and Juba in South Sudan (see under South Sudan, above).

Pakistan: Machar Colony, Karachi

Machar Colony is a large urban slum of over 700,000 inhabitants in Karachi. There is no hospital, just two primary health clinics. The slum has no real services for sanitation or waste disposal. A significant majority of inhabitants are ethnically Bengali.

Saida. A stateless Bengali woman, in her early thirties, born in Pakistan and living in Machar Colony with her seven-year-old son and a brother with mental health problems.

Tanvir. Saida's brother.

Dr. Samina. One of the few doctors working in a community health clinic in Machar Colony.

Preface

Health care is a universal human right—a claim made in speeches and articles describing all the right things about a wonderful world, but a world that seems perpetually out of reach for tens of millions of people. The term *universal* means that everyone, regardless of their citizenship, sex, ethnicity, or national origin, should have access. But that universe, in which health care is a universal right, does not exist. Marginalized groups—such as refugees, internally displaced persons, and the stateless—do not enjoy access to basic health care, in general, or to quality health care, in particular. If they happen to temporarily gain access to care, they are more likely to quickly lose that access than to maintain it.

There are refugees, internally displaced persons, and stateless communities everywhere. They exist in cities that have penthouses promising an expansive view of the ocean, while people stay in camps where water wells dry up within a week after being dug. Some of these marginalized people remain unsettled throughout their lives, living in a perpetual state of transition, moving among communities, cities, states, and countries. Some are born in a slum and stay but are then forced out of health and education services by the political system. In this environment of displacement and exclusion, the likelihood of getting sick is high.

I have often wondered, what do marginalized people do when they are sick and in need? How do these communities access health care in an increasingly nativist world, where the country they live in prioritizes the native inhabitants over them?

Where do they go and whom do they trust?

How do they see the world that does not see them?

There are millions of people who remain invisible to us. They appear as annual statistics in late fall when international organizations estimate the number of forcibly displaced people. Behind the statistics, the human beings remain faceless. Invisibility, however, is itself not equal or homogenous, as some groups are more invisible than others. Consider refugees who have fled to a country that is not a security priority for the rich nations of the world; consider internally displaced persons who are forced to leave their home but cannot cross the border and so remain in their own country as outsiders; and consider stateless persons, those who are outside the strict definition of refugee, so they cannot pursue asylum or citizenship and hence are outside the network of ever-diminishing care and support. And then there are those who come back home, only to find a barren, poisoned, and unfamiliar wasteland.

This book is an attempt to tell their stories.

We Wait for a Miracle

Introduction

My first memories of Islamabad, Pakistan, are of a beautiful, quiet city, seemingly at peace with itself. I was too young to ask questions or worry about social issues. The government at that time, that came to power in a coup in 1977 was controlled by a military establishment, led by General Muhammad Zia-ul-Haq. Life for me and my family was uncomplicated, predictable, and scripted by those in power. It was a bubble; everyone around us was just like us. The schools taught me about the glorious history of our people, the bright future right around the corner, and the never-ending schemes of the evil enemies. All in all, from my vantage point, the society was on a path to progress. There were no serious moral dilemmas or conflicts that needed to be resolved. The government, I was told and taught, was going to take care of all that.

There was, however, one notable exception: the Afghan refugees. People in my bubble, including myself, could not make up our minds whether the refugees coming in from the western border were good or bad. Pakistan, I was told, was the last bastion of freedom against the atheist communists who wanted to reach the warm waters of the

Arabian Sea. This was the prevailing narrative about the Soviet invasion of Afghanistan. Everyone was convinced of this "fact." Many still believe it to be so. The Soviet invasion, we were led to believe, was part of a grand scheme against Pakistan and, by extension, Islam, cooked up in the secretive halls of the Kremlin.

The Afghan war started in 1979 when I was two, but it was peaking at the time of my first memories. There was only one television channel at the time, and it was tightly controlled by the authoritarian state. The evening news was full of endless tales of the valor of the Mujahideen, Islamist resistance groups. The message in our bubble was that, in general, the people of Afghanistan were brave and were standing up to the evil anti-Muslim forces of communism. We were encouraged to support them, as well as everyone from Pakistan who went to Afghanistan to fight evil. This was all good. But then there was a surprising contradiction in private conversations about the Afghans who were now in Pakistan as a consequence of that war.

There was widespread anxiety and hostility toward the poor Afghan refugees, many in Islamabad. I remember being told, at home and in school, that Afghans were responsible for child abductions, that they would take kids away by packing them up in large sacks. There were rumors of Afghan refugees killing children with a hammer. There was a rumor about a new terrorist group named the "Hathora group" (*hathora* means hammer in Urdu).[1] I was told that refugees brought drugs and weapons to destroy our society and that kids who are not doing well in school are most likely struggling because they are spending all their time in snooker and billiard clubs, which were opened and were run by Afghans.

The general feeling in my bubble was that the Afghans were making life hard for the "true" citizens of Pakistan. They were taking jobs from "us," opening stores that sold contraband, and worst of all, they were jumping the queue for US visas. At the very least, they were ungrateful for the generosity of Pakistanis, and more likely they were scheming to take away everything that was good in our lives. I was told to stay away from the Afghans. I was reminded repeatedly that they were not good people. In addition to these unsubstantiated rumors, there was also significant racism toward Pashtuns, who belonged to the same ethnic group as most of the Afghan refugees, especially those who were poor even if they were not technically from Afghanistan. "They are all the same," I remember being told.

But all were not the same. Sometime during the late 1980s, in a relatively new and undeveloped subdivision of Islamabad where my father had built a house in 1985, there was a new grocery store a five-minute walk from our home. The store was run by an Afghan. I do not remember our early interactions with him, but I do remember that it was not long before his was the only store we would go to in the market. He became a friend of our family. Nearly thirty years later, well after I had moved to the United States, I went to his shop during a visit to Islamabad. He remembered me, and we chatted as if time had warped, erasing decades.

Why did our family, and others in the neighborhood, work with him? Why did we consider him almost like family, while other Afghans, people we had never met or interacted with, were blamed for every ill in society? The difference between him and other Afghans was trust. *We trusted him.* I do not know the origins of that trust or the factors that influenced the evolution of that trust, but somehow that trust became an immunity card against prevailing xenophobia.

As Pakistan went through stages of political turmoil, chaos, coups, and episodes of violence, the public sphere separated the "good" Afghans from the "bad" ones. The prevailing sense today, as it was back then, is that most Afghans are bad, scheming, and ungrateful, and a few are not.

This lack of trust between the people and the refugees manifests itself not only in daily interactions and perceptions but in services, including access to health care.

The fundamental premise of this book is that while there are important contextual differences between countries and communities, there are central aspects to how health care is navigated and negotiated. The communities do not have to be in geographic proximity, or have cultural ties to each other, or be driven out of the system by the same crisis (whether it be war or economic collapse or climate change or a natural disaster), but their experience, at a fundamental level, is influenced by a series of similar factors that cut across cultures, countries, and institutions.

I've chosen to introduce the reader to these aspects through the personal stories of three actual people, from three different countries and communities, who have tried to navigate their local health care system. These up-close stories show how the health care systems actually work and, unfortunately, how they don't. Three people—Rafael, Henry, and Saida—represent communities facing real challenges, challenges that are often outside of our view. Few in academia, and even fewer in the media, focus on the stateless, those who return, or the ones who are driven out not because of conflict but because of economic collapse of the state. Their stories are often too complicated, less exciting, and harder to associate with a linear narrative. Yet, in many ways, their stories also represent realities we choose to ignore, even when we are researching the health challenges of refugees and internally displaced persons (IDPs) in better-studied communities. As we'll see, our inability to provide adequate care is not simply because of lack of funds; it is also because of our own biases, racism, and ill-will.

During the research for this book, which lasted several years, I met dozens of people. First I met people in-person and, when that was no longer possible due to COVID-19 travel restrictions, I spoke to people via WhatsApp and phone calls. These included individuals who were living in camps and informal settlements, as well as caregivers, workers at nongovernmental organizations (NGOs), and doctors, nurses, and lawyers working in the community. I spoke to lab technicians and to construction workers building new health care centers. I spent time with pharmacists and with spiritual healers. In addition, I met many remarkable individuals early on in my research—and I wanted to tell their stories—but I couldn't stay connected with them because they were repeatedly forced to flee. This was particularly true in Yemen, where the internally displaced communities that I was working with were often on the move and had very real reasons to lay low and avoid communication.

Pivotal factors influencing access to health care

In communities of forcibly displaced persons, access to health care remains fragile and a source of great anxiety. The basis for this anxiety is not only the physical pain associated with illness but also the emotional toll associated with the loss of their meager resources and the fear of harassment and persecution. From my research and interactions with individuals and communities, I have identified three pivotal, interdependent factors that influence access to health care by marginalized groups: the presence (or absence) of trust between the patient and the provider, an organic and dynamic social network that is the basis of information and financial support for the forcibly displaced, and a government regulatory environment.

The first factor is *trust*. Those who are forcibly displaced go to institutions and providers whom they can trust. This does not mean that every institution or provider they go to is one that enjoys their trust. It simply means that members of these communities will go to great lengths, and even take substantial risks, to seek care from those they trust. This also means that they are wary of going to other institutions, even if this means delaying essential care, if they feel that they cannot trust the individual and institution to safeguard their well-being. Communities can be distrustful of individuals and institutions because they may feel a strong sense of pervasive racism and exclusion.

Trust is bidirectional in accessing health services. Refugees may choose to not go to a place they do not trust, and the state may only offer services to those they trust. Access to health care is also at the mercy of the power dynamic between those who control the resources and those who seek basic services, which creates a parallel universe of access.

In states like Pakistan, with a large population but a small budget for health care (the public education budget is even smaller), and with little accountability in the administration of those funds, individual hospitals and staff persons have a great deal of power over who gets served. Unfortunately, Pakistan's case—a weak public health system, political strife, and large number of migrants—is not unusual. It is seen in numerous low- and middle-income countries in Asia, Africa and South America.

The second pivotal factor that influences access to health care is an organic *social network*. The social network, whether through digital apps and Facebook or through word of mouth or memory, is a resource both for information and for actual financial means to seek care. The social network can also enhance or diminish trust in the system, institutions, and organizations.

The third pivotal factor influencing access to quality care is the *regulatory environment*. When the government shuts its doors to the vulnerable, they look elsewhere for care and evaluate what is accessible. Private sector doctors and hospitals could be an option in theory, but they are often prohibitively expensive. Since the refugees, IDPs, and stateless communities often have limited financial capacity, they seek care in the shadows of the system. They find illegal providers, who benefit from the vulnerability of these communities. Counterfeit drug sellers or untrained and unlicensed medical professionals are able to exploit those in need. Unfortunately, unlicensed and illegal providers are not just high risk but also cannot be brought to justice if things go wrong. Government policies can crack down on black markets, illegal providers, and counterfeiters; and even if the government still provides few avenues for accessing the public system, the demand for care can create an opportunity for NGOs and licensed providers to fill that niche.

In addition to the personal stories of actual people, this book includes in-depth discussions of issues around marginalized communities accessing health care in a variety of countries. Each chapter begins with short sections about each main character—Rafael, Henry, and Saida—followed by a longer section analyzing the topic.

Chapter 1 describes the current situation of marginalized communities—who they are and where they live. Chapter 2 focuses on a brief history of refugees and refugee camps with an eye toward health care access in those camps. Chapter 3 introduces the reader to the two models of health care systems: a separate system used only by displaced persons versus one national system for both citizens and displaced persons. Chapter 4 looks at how marginalized communities use social networks to navigate health care systems.

Chapter 5 describes the many unregulated practices for selling medicines and medical procedures, and who the providers are in this underground market. Chapter 6 looks at the benefits and challenges of digital technologies in accessing health care. Finally, chapter 7 shows that racism and discrimination are significant barriers to accessing health care for displaced persons.

Chapter 1
Current Situations of Forcibly Displaced Persons

Rafael flees from Venezuela

The thing that Rafael missed the most was not being able to lift his daughter Christina. He missed laughing when she sat on his shoulders, screaming with delight, as he ran, jumped, and swayed. She'd hang on by clasping her arms around his neck. Christina was his youngest, and she would turn nine in a month. Rafael had missed her last two birthdays, and he'd likely miss this one as well.

The last week had been especially hard, as Rafael had been unable to talk to Christina. The Wi-Fi in the room he was renting was not working very well. "Too many people are getting on the Wi-Fi," the landlady told him. The apartment building was in a dense part of Bogotá, Colombia, with many apartment buildings, and each apartment had many people. He rented a room within the apartment of a distant family member. On the other side of the border, Christina waited for his calls, but her Wi-Fi was not much better. Last week, the connection had collapsed completely.

The other thing Rafael missed was the air of his Venezuelan hometown of Complejo Turistico El Morro, Lecheria, in the Anzoategui Province, right on the Caribbean Sea and to the east of Caracas. It was always warm, breezy, colorful, and teeming with people from across the world. Rafael's friends had families in Italy, Lebanon, Spain, and Portugal. Lately Chinese workers and businessmen had arrived to make this coastal city their home, and new Chinese eateries were the latest addition to the long list of excellent restaurants in the city.

Rafael had worked as a lawyer in Venezuela before he became a jobless migrant in another country. His work had focused on financial transactions and mergers and acquisitions. He'd had an array of clients that ranged from housing societies, banks, companies, and individuals who needed him to resolve a financial lawsuit. A few years earlier, his work had started to become more difficult. Since 2014, the economy had been in freefall, and the financial crisis had enveloped the whole society. The government of Venezuela, led by Nicolás Maduro since 2013, facing a weakening support among its base, was trying to wrest control of institutions it felt were not bending to its will. During the early days of the economic crisis, Rafael represented a housing society that was providing legal support to its residents. The government had been trying hard, and unsuccessfully, to take control of the housing society under the guise of Gran Misión Vivienda (the Great Housing Mission).[1] The Great Mission was envisioned as a populist project, designed to create public housing for the urban working class. In reality it meant forcibly taking control of existing, privately owned housing. Rafael represented a housing society and its investments, and for a few years he had successfully kept the government at bay.

Then came August 2017. Rafael's daughters were on vacation with their mother on Margarita Island, 150 kilometers north of Lecheria. It was the last day of the month, a Thursday, and Rafael was having lunch with a friend at his mother-in-law's home. The weather was excellent, and the breeze was cool. In the middle of his lunch, his phone buzzed. Rafael looked at his phone and saw that the call was from a friend.

Rafael didn't pick up, but he made a mental note to call his friend after lunch. The phone buzzed again. It was the same friend. Rafael again declined the call. The phone rang one more time, and finally Rafael picked up.

"Your arrest orders have been issued." The friend was speaking in a hushed, anxious voice. His friend worked in the courts and thus had inside information.

"What?" Rafael asked, unsure what to make of this.

"The government will be sending police to arrest you. You need to leave immediately. The order is coming directly from the attorney general."

Situations like this were not unheard of. In fact, they were becoming more and more common. Rafael had read about them in the papers and on social media, and he'd personally known some people who'd been picked up recently by the government. Most were never heard from again. He'd never thought of himself as someone important. He'd never thought they would come for him.

Rafael's friend told him that his bank accounts, including his credit cards, were frozen. (Later, Rafael would learn that the government had also ordered the auctioning of his personal property, including his house.) His friend recommended that Rafael escape as fast as he could because he was certain the government was tracking Rafael. Right before he hung up, Rafael's friend had three final pieces of advice: "Don't go back to your home. Turn off your phone. And take the battery out."

Rafael had to hide immediately and, to survive, leave the country. He was shaken, unsure, and initially even skeptical of what was going on. But his friend was insistent, almost pleading. Rafael knew this friend was well connected and his sources were reliable. He also knew his friend was sincere. As much as the friend was trustworthy, the government was not.

Rafael left lunch abruptly, found a taxi, and decided to go into hiding. Using the taxi driver's phone, he called another friend, Nicolas, and told him that he needed to stay with him for a few days, maybe more. Nicolas immediately agreed and did not ask any questions.

Rafael's daughters were out of town, so there was no need to tell them why he wasn't coming home. No one knew where Rafael was except for a few close friends, who immediately started planning his escape out of Venezuela. One friend, Sophia, went to Rafael's home and packed a small suitcase of clothes: underwear for five days, two flannel shirts, four short-sleeved shirts, and two pairs of jeans. She didn't bother to pack a sweater.

Another friend, Oscar, had a cousin who worked for airport security. Oscar asked his cousin for a favor. He only told him that there would be a person, who was wanted by the government, coming to the airport, and this person was like a brother to Oscar. The cousin's job was to ensure that the person could pass airport security without any questions. Oscar knew his cousin could be trusted and that he was equally frustrated by the government and its rampant corruption, even though he worked for airport security, which was in essence the state. (Oscar never told Rafael whether there was any money exchanged between him and his cousin. Rafael never asked.)

Oscar told Rafael to arrive at the airport around midday on September 1, when some workers would be off for lunch. The flight out of Venezuela was going to depart around six o'clock in the evening. Oscar calculated that six hours would be enough time for Rafael to get through the maze of security and catch his flight.

Rafael did as he was told and, even though he didn't have a ticket in hand or specific information about the flight, showed up at the airport on time. Oscar's cousin was there to help him quietly slip through security. A couple of policemen were standing there. They gave Rafael a slight nod and then hid him in different parts of the airport before eventually getting him inside the terminal.

On the other side of security, there was another man waiting for Rafael. This man, whose name Rafael never asked, handed Rafael a ticket. On that particular afternoon, there weren't many flights leaving Lecheria, but there was one to Guayaquil, a port city in Ecuador. Rafael looked at his ticket and found that he held not one but two tickets. The second one, stapled to the first, was for a flight from Guayaquil to Bogotá, the capital of Colombia.

Over the last decade, Colombia's relationship with Venezuela had become tenuous, as the two countries adopted different political ideologies.[2] With those ideologies came new friends and enemies, and new investments. Bogotá was not just the capital of a neighboring country; it was the place where many Venezuelans, including distant relatives of Rafael, lived and worked in a variety of sectors.

Rafael waited quietly. He never turned on his phone, and he kept the phone and the battery in two different pockets. He had not spoken to his daughters in a few days, and he desperately wanted to call them and tell them that everything would be okay and that they should not worry. He wanted to place a video call and see Christina before he boarded his flight. Despite the strong urge and despite twice coming close to calling her, he somehow fought the urge and did not take the risk. Rafael still remembers those moments waiting for the flight as the most anxious of his life.

His first flight was on time. His heart was pounding as he got in line to board. As he handed the ticket to the agent at the gate, his palms became sweaty. Rafael waited for the agent to ask a question that would upend his escape plans and take him to the authorities. Instead, the agent stamped the ticket with a mechanical motion of her hand. She never looked up.

Rafael, still unsure of what was going on, reached his seat and stowed his small suitcase. During the flight Rafael kept to himself—he didn't look out the window at his beloved city or talk to the passenger next to him. The flight landed in Guayaquil, and Rafael felt a temporary sense of relief but the anxiety was still palpable. It was eight o'clock at night, local time. His next flight was scheduled for four o'clock the next morning. During the wait, Rafael, anxious and worried, kept to himself and nervously stared at a clock, which seemed to turn so slowly that Rafael was certain it was frozen.

The flight from Guayaquil to Bogotá wasn't much better. He remained tense, almost taut, for the entire flight. Though Rafael had not eaten anything in nearly twenty-four hours, he still couldn't eat on the plane. He took a few sips from the can of Coke handed to him. The flight eventually landed in Bogotá.

Standing in line for immigration, Rafael knew that something could still go wrong, and he could be deported. As he reached the counter and presented his passport to get stamped, the immigration agent did not have any questions for Rafael.

As Rafael stepped out of the airport terminal in Bogotá, he was wearing a short-sleeved shirt. It was cold, only a few degrees Celsius (around 45 degrees Fahrenheit). Coming from a warm, breezy environment, he was utterly unprepared for the cold. With no sweater in his suitcase, he instead wore multiple layers and a flannel shirt over his short sleeves to keep warm. The air felt heavy. He could smell diesel, a near-permanent feature of Bogotá's air.

He looked back, in the direction of what he thought was Venezuela, unsure of when he'd see Christina again.

Henry's brother leaves his Ugandan refugee camp

Henry gazed down the road toward Uganda. His eyes traced the pathway and imagined its far end. The road wasn't in good shape, but it was the only one that went to his brother. Henry pictured the road, alternating between asphalt and dirt, starting at his feet and winding its way through towns and villages from here in Malakan, South Sudan, more than 200 kilometers to the Bidi Bidi refugee camp in Uganda. Henry knew the road like the back of his hand on the South Sudanese side, but he'd never made the journey to Uganda.

He had seen pictures and heard all kinds of stories about Bidi Bidi, his brother's home for the past four years. It was a sprawling camp that was among the largest in the world.[3] Henry was told that it was a world unto itself—with its own hierarchy, rules, commerce, and corruption. It had all the players he was familiar with: NGOs and locals, government and army, and of course lots and lots of intermediary people, all in there for a cut of the profit and control. He knew that people had started their own businesses there and were now employing others. For Henry, the place sounded too chaotic. He was not cut out for a place like that. Unlike his brother Solomon and others in the family, Henry had never moved to Bidi Bidi nor had even considered visiting. As a nurse and as a pastor, he'd found his professional and spiritual calling on this side of the border: in his village and in his country.

Henry was now incredibly busy after receiving a voice message on his phone from his brother.

"Coming next week," the message said.

This had been developing for some time. Solomon, who'd spent years in the camp, increasingly felt lost, confused, and harassed. He could no longer live in Bidi Bidi.

"No more camp, but home," Solomon told Henry.

Home? Henry wondered what that meant for Solomon.

Henry had grown up in the village of Malakan, home to a few thousand people. (Outsiders often confuse Malakan with Malakal, a large city of over a hundred thousand people, a few hundred kilometers to the north.) Malakan had a single store, which served as a grocery store, a drug store, and a butcher shop. Henry personally knew the owner and went there often. To the owner, Henry was a supplier of goods, a trader, a customer, a benefactor, and a spiritual guide.

Decades ago, Henry's ancestors had made Malakan home, cultivating and herding goats. Goat-herding was a trade Henry learned early in his life and one he would return to time and time again, especially when all other means of earning a living failed. Born in 1969, Henry showed strong interest in studying, though he was not bad at herding either. When he was in his early teens, Henry insisted to his father that he wanted to study beyond what was available in their village. So, Henry went to a middle school in Wonduruba, a town located a few kilometers from Malakan. Though it was nearby, and accessible on foot and a bicycle, it was a place starkly different from Malakan. The roads were better, and some houses were made out of stone, brick, or concrete rather than the dried mud and thatched roofs of Malakan. Henry commuted between Malakan and Wonduruba for his primary and secondary school years. After he finished his intermediate school, there were no more options in Malakan or in Wonduruba. If he wanted to study further, he'd have to go outside the region.

In 1985 he moved to Juba, a city 130 kilometers away that later became the capital of South Sudan. This was a time of the second civil war in the region; the first war went from 1955 to 1972.[4] The tensions in the region had been simmering for a while, but this was more than the routine skirmishes. On one side was the South Sudanese People's Liberation Movement, and on the other was the well-equipped Sudanese army comprised of officers and soldiers largely from the north. The war soon reached small towns. Life was disrupted with chaos, checkpoints, and frequent reports of torture.

At some point, traveling was too dangerous, so Henry couldn't return to Malakan but had to stay in Juba. Casualties were everywhere. While Henry's parents survived and were able to stay in their home, his cousins, aunts, and uncles were forced out of their homes and were displaced. As the months and years passed, there were new treaties, new coalitions, and new coups.[5] Even when things looked fine from a distance, they weren't good on the ground. It was years before Henry could return to Malakan and see his home. Those were hard days for Henry. He felt alone, frustrated, anxious, and angry.

Like many others who were trying to find meaning in their lives, Henry found comfort and direction in the church. Henry was smart, inquisitive, thoughtful, and hardworking. He also had the ability to explain things plainly, and people gravitated toward him. He had been active in his Anglican church since childhood. Henry's pastor in Juba noticed his abilities and encouraged him to consider becoming a minister. Henry felt inspired by this confidence from his mentor and pastor. He enrolled in a program at the Bishop Gwynne College to become an ordained minister. For several years, the church consumed all of his time. In 1995 he was ordained as a deacon, and in 1996 he became a fully ordained priest.

Henry had planned to be away from his Malakan home for a couple of years; it took him nearly twenty years to return and settle (temporarily) in Malakan. During that time, much had changed, both in Malakan and in Henry's outlook of the wider world. Continued conflicts had wiped out entire villages, torched homes, and created new enemies and newer allies. When he was away, Henry had heard the stories of torture and brutality. Now, at home, he saw for himself the horrors of open and infected wounds. He saw women who had been raped and men who were on the verge of suicide. His church was full of orphans, who were often sick and always hungry.

Surrounded by this chaos and misery, Henry was becoming increasingly restless. He knew that he was ordained to be a man of the cloth, but Henry now felt that he had received a second calling. This voice from inside was as convincing as the first one that had persuaded him to become a pastor. Like the first one, this one was about healing. But it was a lot more literal this time. Henry went back to school in 2000 and enrolled in a health sciences program in Juba. The program wasn't free, but Henry was resourceful and frugal. He made it work. Being good with his hands, he also picked up skills as a lab technician, which allowed him to earn extra money (he wasn't paid as well as a nurse, nor as a minister). However, he still didn't earn enough as a technician, so Henry did what people in his family had done for hundreds of years. He also herded goats in Malakan. After finishing his health sciences training, Henry found employment at the hospital in Juba. He still worked at his church and kept his goats.

In the early 2000s things were changing rapidly in the region. There were new peace deals, new-power sharing agreements, and new warlords. Above all, there was on-the-ground support for a new, independent state. Then in January 2011 there was a referendum on whether

South Sudan should become independent. Henry voted yes. So did everyone in his church. Seven months later in July, a new state was born.

Henry clearly remembers that day and the excitement, even in his small village. People stayed up all night, excited. Yet the euphoria was short lived. The peace, which people believed would be a consequence of statehood and independence, did not materialize.

A series of events ruined that dream shared by millions. First there was a war between the new country and its northern neighbor, Sudan. But worse was yet to come in the form of a civil war. The new president of South Sudan and his vice president had a falling out, prompting the vice president to go into exile and mount an armed rebellion.[6] For Henry, this war was much closer to home. There was active, house-to-house fighting in Malakan. Henry was living and working in Juba at that time, but he regularly visited Malakan. His older brother Solomon was living in Malakan with his family, and Solomon's family got caught up in the war. A rumor spread in the village that Solomon was working for the government and had picked up arms and fought against the militia led by the former vice president. The village had recently come under the control of the anti-government militia, and there were house-to-house searches for anyone not loyal to their cause. Solomon was warned of the searches and ran away, barely in time to save his life. But there was little else he could save. In an attack on his village, Solomon's animals were taken away, and his land and house were torched.

Angry, dejected, and without a home or a means to support himself or his family, Solomon suffered a stroke. Henry, despite being a nurse, could do little to help. Henry did not have any training in treating mental health issues and had no medicines he could give to his brother. Henry's best advice to his brother was to seek help in Uganda in the camps for displaced South Sudanese people. Henry had heard that the NGOs there had resources to treat strokes and other disorders. Solomon was initially reluctant and did not want to leave home, but as his condition deteriorated further, he eventually agreed.

In early 2016 Solomon, with his family, traveled the single road from Malakan to Uganda. He moved to a new land with a new status: *refugee.*

Solomon and his family were part of the caravan that went south. Such caravans were becoming the norm.[7] At the border, Solomon was registered at a big, white tent. Depressed, Solomon barely spoke. His wife spoke for him. There was an initial health check, but nothing was recorded about his stroke or his mental state. The line was long, and the caregiver had to register many people. Solomon and his family were given rations for a month, and then they were moved to Bidi Bidi, a place with endless tents, shacks, and huts made by people like Solomon. No one from the camp administration came and checked up on Solomon the next day or the next week or the next month. In this settlement, far away from home, they were mostly on their own.

Solomon stayed for years. With time, his condition worsened. He was quiet most of the time, and when he wasn't speaking, he was angry, anxious, and sometimes violent. He frequently complained of headaches or pains in his chest. He talked about seeing things no one else could see. He was all alone in his struggles. In the chaotic and cutthroat world of Bidi Bidi, where only the fittest could survive, Solomon had no chance.

Henry was in touch with his brothers' family through people in the camp who knew Henry through his tribe or his church. As mobile phones became more common, there were calls and then voice messages. New economies grew out of the misery of people like Solomon through intermediaries and entrepreneurs who would transport items between Malakan and Bidi Bidi. They would take a big cut for this transport, but as a minister, Henry received a special rate in return for praying for the person.

Henry had one advantage. He had recently started working at a larger hospital in Juba as a lab technician. It was a job that paid better than being a nurse at a smaller hospital, and he would occasionally receive donations of medications from the hospital. Mostly the drugs were for malaria, other infections, or fever control, but every now and then, he'd receive drugs to treat mental health disorders. Henry was unfamiliar with many of the brands and did not know the right dose, but he believed something given to Solomon was better than nothing. Henry would collect donations until he had a decent amount to last Solomon a few months. Then he'd wrap them carefully and send them to Solomon via someone going to Uganda.

The medicines were a lifeline for Solomon, but the donations were sporadic and there were long periods when Henry wasn't given any. In those times, desperate for anything, Solomon would buy the medicines in the black market that thrived in Bidi Bidi. Cash was always preferred, but Solomon and his family had none. So they had to pay in oil or grains—precious rations they got from the aid agencies. Medicines for Solomon meant he would be calm and not violent. But it meant there was less food for the family.

The family had come to terms with its fate and had learned to live in the system of corruption, barter, and continuous food insecurity. Then in March 2020, COVID-19 hit Uganda. The government—800 kilometers to the south in Kampala—decided to impose a lockdown that impacted every part of the country,[8] including Bidi Bidi. Overnight, military trucks appeared, and soldiers, wearing poorly fitting green uniforms, waved their big guns and shouted from maskless faces to ensure that there was strict compliance in the camp. Initially Solomon and his family were provided food, but then that too disappeared. All of a sudden, the likelihood of survival in the camp decreased sharply. Overnight, the informal economy and barter trade collapsed and threatened the lives of refugees in Uganda.[9] Rumors took hold in the camp, about the government using COVID-19 to send the refugees back to South Sudan. The feeling of helplessness was palpable in the air.[10] One of Solomon's friends took his own life.

The sense of loss gave rise to a new sentiment: maybe South Sudan was not so bad after all or at least not as bad as Bidi Bidi in times of COVID-19. The idea to go back home started to take shape among many families in Bidi Bidi.

When Solomon told his family that he wanted to return to Malakan, no one stopped him. Convinced that it was the right thing to do, Solomon recorded a voice message for Henry.

"Coming home," he said.

Saida lives permanently in a Pakistan camp as a stateless Bengali

Home—a strange word for a cramped place where Saida has lived all her life except for the one year she was married. Home was a one-room place with concrete walls, badly painted years ago with cheap, pastel-colored paint. Not much paint was left, and the unsmooth walls were now an unpleasant combination of streaks of faded and peeled paint, black dust, gray concrete, and the reddish-orange remnant of bricks.

This one-room dwelling was occupied by Saida and her mother, her brother, and her seven-year-old son. In theory, Saida's home was close to the sea. There was a time, she had been told, when you could smell the salt of the Arabian Sea in the evening breeze. Saida had never experienced that. Now, with new constructions, heaps of trash, and the land that was being reclaimed, it was not even possible to see the sea. There was no longer any smell of salt in the air, no breeze in the evening, no lullaby of the sea at night. Those things happened only in books, which were not available in her neighborhood.

The neighborhood where Saida lived was called Machar Colony. It was home to over 700,000 people,[11] most of whom like Saida were ethnically Bengali. They were poor, stateless, and largely absent within the national discourse. As far as the government of Pakistan was concerned, she did not exist. Neither did her mother, her brother, nor her son. Nor had her late father existed. Saida had no identity documents, was not in any database, and was explicitly not counted in any national census.

Saida was born in Machar Colony and had spent her entire life in this sprawling environment. Like an organism, the colony had grown, seemingly in a random manner, in all directions, including toward the sea. Built as a small fishing village in the 1960s on the southeastern edge of Karachi,[12] her ancestors had come here in the early 1970s.

Saida's ancestors were ethnically Bengali, hailing from the eastern wing of a two-part Pakistan. In 1947, when the British colonial rule ended in India, two new countries emerged, India and Pakistan. Pakistan, in 1947, was not a geographically contiguous territory but two areas of land on either side of India. The larger area, on the western side of India, was West Pakistan, and the smaller but more populated area, on the eastern side of India, was called East Pakistan. Most people in East Pakistan spoke Bangla and shared a strong sense of cultural identity associated with the language. Soon after the partition of India, a feeling of resentment among the Bengalis in East Pakistan started to take hold. It was fueled by injustice, xenophobia, and racism from the western part of the country, which enjoyed the seat of the government, dominance in the military, and the majority of the bureaucracy.

The Bangla-speaking East Pakistan was producing jute, a cash crop at the time, but the proceeds from those exports were largely going to West Pakistan. There was also a systematic attack on the language, culture, and heritage of the Bangla-speaking community. They were considered inferior and less-devout Muslims.[13] Political decisions, internal allocation of funds, and development efforts favored West Pakistan, while East Pakistan continued to suffer economically. After nearly a quarter century of an unhappy and fractious partnership, things came to a head in 1971 when a civil war culminated in the break-up of East and West Pakistan and the creation of a new country. There was no more East Pakistan. It was now Bangladesh.

In the chaos of the civil war, and with hopes of a better future, many low-income Bengalis migrated to West Pakistan, which was economically more prosperous and (at that time) offered prospects for a better future. The western half was now known simply as Pakistan. The economically distressed Bengalis settled in shanties around the Arabian Sea in Karachi where there was demand for cheap labor for fishermen and shrimp peelers.

Before 1971, Bengalis living in East Pakistan were citizens of Pakistan (albeit not treated as well as their compatriots in West Pakistan). This meant that they could travel from Dhaka in the east to Karachi in the west just as easily as they could travel from city to city within East Pakistan. In the chaotic period during and immediately after the 1971 war, there was confusion and a general lack of clarity about allowed movement between the two parts.

As Saida's ancestors moved from a poor suburb of Dhaka to Karachi, in their minds they were simply moving from one part of their country to the other. In the eyes of the state of Pakistan, these people were not citizens but were outsiders coming into a separate sovereign country. They had no government-issued documentation to prove they had migrated to Pakistan legally or were ever citizens of Pakistan. After the bloody episode of 1971, it was impossible to go back and get documents, if there were even any documents in the first place. Many people who made the move had paid intermediaries and smugglers, traveled through a hazardous terrain, and boarded overcrowded boats.[14] There were no receipts of travel showing origin, destination, or the means of travel, such as the name of the vessel.

Poverty, illiteracy, and xenophobia against Bengalis created an exclusionary environment in Pakistan. To politicians and the military in Pakistan, these people were either the enemy themselves or at least enemy sympathizers. They were viewed as those who had helped break the country into two, and therefore they did not deserve any rights or privileges. Such sentiment has continued for the last five decades.[15] The accepted view was that if they could not be sent back (since there was no appetite to accept poor, illiterate, and unskilled persons by the new state of Bangladesh), then they should at least be viewed with suspicion.

Saida's family, like hundreds of thousands of others, decided to stick together, hoping that the state would take notice of their large numbers and do something about their statelessness. These Bengalis in Karachi considered themselves Pakistani not Bangladeshi.

Machar Colony continued to grow.[16] It was a place where other Bengalis lived under the radar, or perhaps under the watchful eye of the state, which didn't accept them but at least tolerated them. Over time, it was not just Bengalis who came to live there but also other marginalized communities who had nowhere else to go. Not everyone had crossed India to come to this part of Pakistan. Some were coming from much shorter distances. This was the last stop before the sea.

A haphazard structure of houses emerged.[17] A maze of streets and its own economy soon followed. But life here was hard and outside the domain of rights provided by the state. The state did not invest in sanitation, housing, education, or health services. It was not a well-organized housing community to begin with, but over time it became a slum with one of the worst urban environments in the city. There was trash, sewage, stagnant water, and dust, making it a health hazard for the community. Plastic bottles and bags became ubiquitous, dotting the land, and covering what little drainage there was. The first rain of monsoon season brought stagnant water, which became a permanent feature of the landscape. Additional rains led to flooded streets that also contained trash and sewage.[18]

Saida had grown up with trash in the streets, but the amount had progressively increased. So did the diseases. Skin diseases were common among the shrimp peelers; respiratory diseases and cough were a routine among children; and people increasingly complained of stomach ailments.

All day long, children of all ages played in the streets of trash and wastewater. Not everyone went to the few schools in the community. In the world outside Machar Colony, there were public schools for children, but obtaining admission to these schools required identification documents, a rare and prized possession. Without any formal papers, the majority of Bengalis could not enroll their children in the state schools.[19] Private schools were often too expensive, and even if the children somehow managed to get into a private primary school with the help of a sympathetic school administrator, the secondary schools were far stricter about identification. Being admitted to the national exam for secondary school without formal identification was next to impossible. Trying your luck at school admission meant taking a risk. What if the school administrators tipped off the police about you? The police in Karachi, notorious for permanently working in the gray zone between law and lawlessness, would either demand a hefty bribe or would turn you over to law enforcement authorities. For girls, any interaction with police was certain to end in harassment or worse. Everyone around Saida lived in a permanent state of anxiety.

Saida grew up in a community that was shaped by a *disincentive* to go to school and an incentive to earn money. There was a continuous demand for shrimp peelers, and the employer did not care if you were educated or not, if you were five or fifty-five. The earnings, while paltry, were guaranteed in the harvesting season. The work was back-breaking and done in overcrowded spaces, full of pain and a near-constant exposure to skin disease that would go untreated because no one could see a doctor. But there was no other way to put food on the table.

Saida's family became part of the same business that everyone around them was involved in. Saida started peeling shrimp when she was five. Everyone around her did the same. In this toxic mixture of poverty, frustration, and discrimination, drug dealers found fertile ground. By the time Saida grew up, addiction was rampant.[20] As was domestic abuse. Saida saw it firsthand with her own father, who was an addict who abused her mother every night. She saw it with her neighbor and her cousins. Like the permanent state of poverty, it was part of the colony's DNA and its architecture. So was early marriage. Saida's life was no exception.

Forcibly displaced persons: Who they are and where they live

By early 2022, there were nearly 100 million displaced persons globally.[21] Eighteen months earlier, the number was 80 million.[22] This data, updated annually by the United Nations High Commissioner for Refugees (UNHCR), has been produced almost every year since 1951,[23] but only recently has there been more publicity around it.

The focus of UNHCR has not always been global.[24] It was formed in the aftermath of the Second World War, and its original focus was almost exclusively Europe.[25] More specifically, its mandate was to help and assist refugees from Europe only and, more narrowly, only those who had been forced to leave their homes before January 1, 1951. This meant that millions of refugees in other parts of the world including Africa, South Asia, the Middle East, and Latin America didn't receive help from the agency for its first sixteen years in existence. This deliberate exclusion included people in Pakistan.[26] This changed in 1967 when UNHCR expanded its mandate to include refugees outside Europe.[27]

Today, the number of displaced persons reported is used extensively by international aid agencies, humanitarian organizations, and academics, but it comes with its own set of assumptions. Many suggest that this number is *unprecedented* and that we are now living in a time in human history when the greatest number of people have been displaced from their homes. There is little historical evidence to back this claim.[28] Conservative estimates suggest that as many as 200 million (nearly twice the number used by UNHCR today) were displaced during the Second World War alone. Half of those were internally displaced within China at various stages of the war.

The fixation on the number and recent episodes of global displacement also suggests that the current crises are somehow the worst episodes of forced displacement in history. This claim also stands on thin ground. The partition of British India led to the migration of nearly 15 million displaced persons between India and (what was to become) Pakistan.[29] This number is greater than the current combined number of displaced persons in Somalia, Afghanistan, and Syria, and the Rohingya refugees in Bangladesh.

Beyond the historical inaccuracies, there are statistical problems with the single number that is often quoted in the news. The number estimated by UNHCR reflects both refugees—those who cross international borders—and internally displaced persons (IDPs), those who are forced from their homes but do not leave the geographic boundaries of their country. This composite statistic consists of one-third refugees and two-thirds IDPs.[30] There is however a problem when the current statistic is compared against historical data. The number of IDPs has only been collected since the 1990s when UNHCR expanded its mandate to include IDPs.[31] Therefore any comparison to the past would be inaccurate since it would not have included IDPs. Furthermore, the IDP statistics are often biased[32] and based on self-reporting by governments. A government that is responsible for creating an IDP crisis in the first place may have myriad reasons to underreport, or inflate, the number of IDPs based on their political or economic interests.

Beyond the historical issues with statistics, there are other problems with the general perception of who is a displaced person (*refugee* is often used as an umbrella term in mass media, and few distinctions are made between refugees, internally displaced or stateless persons) and how that individual is presented to a broader audience. Most news stories about refugees often create a uniform image. Even though, each year additional stories about humanitarian crises are told (often synchronized with the release of the UNHCR number or in response to a new crisis), the image of who the refugee is often disconnected from reality. The news stories, and public attention, are also quick to move to the next crisis while previous ones are forgotten. For example, in light of the crisis in Afghanistan in 2021, few reports referred to the Rohingya people, and even fewer referred to the Syrians. Reports on South Sudanese are hard to find, and the Palestinian refugees are only mentioned in the news during an armed conflict involving Palestine and Israel.

Refugees

In general, refugees are shown to be people who are driven out of their homes due to war (mostly civil war between the government and "rebels"), are housed in large refugee camps, and are taken care of by international (mostly UN-affiliated) or humanitarian agencies. Various celebrities[33] who get their pictures taken in these camps further reinforce the image of a hapless refugee in a refugee camp in need of support from Western benefactors. The crisis, which displaced the person and created refugees, is painted as one that was somewhat unpredictable and sudden (e.g., the sudden withdrawal of US troops in Afghanistan in mid-August 2021), despite strong evidence for the persistent and long-standing underlying political, financial, and social issues.[34] Thus the presented image disconnects the crisis from the broader historical trends. Little attention is paid to social injustice, corruption, autocratic rulers, or outside interference from powerful states that led to the crisis. Finally, the images created in print, electronic, and social media fail to capture the reality that some of those forced to leave their homes have been (or will be) displaced for decades,[35] rather than being in the camp for only a transitory period, as if they were victims of a natural disaster like a hurricane or an earthquake.

While all the elements painted in the typical, monochromatic image may be individually present in several crises that have forced people out of their homes, a one-dimensional image is incomplete and often inaccurate. It also creates a response strategy that is insufficient and ineffective, as it fails to understand and address the systems-level issues or is disconnected from history.

Internally Displaced Persons

Not all displaced communities will cross international borders, and therefore will not become refugees. In fact, the majority of those who are forcibly displaced do not leave the geographic borders of their country. Internal displacement, defined as forced movement of people within the borders of their own country, constitutes a significant majority of communities that are forced out of their homes.[36] Civil wars, sometimes spanning decades, create communities that face perpetual violence and hence are forced to move. In Colombia, for example, there are nearly six million IDPs, one of the largest numbers worldwide.[37] The IDPs in Colombia are on the move because of violence faced by communities all across the country during a decades-long war between the government and Revolutionary Armed Forces of Colombia (FARC). Despite multiple peace treaties, millions of people are forced to abandon their homes due to continued armed violence, loss of property, lack of social integration programs, and high levels of unemployment.[38]

For IDPs worldwide, there are several reasons not to cross international borders, including the lack of any viable way to cross. For example, Yemeni citizens caught in the conflict led by Saudi Arabia and allies on one side and Houthi groups on the other have nowhere to go because the nearest, largest, and most viable border is with Saudi Arabia, where Yemeni refugees are not welcome. Yemen's other border, with Oman, is on the far east side of the country, which makes it too far to travel for some; in addition, the Omani government has little desire to receive Yemeni citizens fleeing for their safety. Caught in this conflict, Yemeni citizens are forced to stay within their country; some families have had to move from one village or settlement to another several times in the last five years.[39] Alternatively, for some displaced communities, the nearest international border may be with a state that itself is dealing with political instability or conflict. Internally displaced persons from northwest Pakistan in the mid-2000s[40] were unwilling to travel to Afghanistan because of its lack of political and financial stability.

Stateless Persons

A third category of displaced persons are stateless persons, who are often perpetually displaced. Some stateless persons, due to conflict or persecution, may be forced to move to a new and unwelcoming state that does not give them a right to seek asylum or does not consider them a refugee, while simultaneously their previous country strips them of citizenship or refuses to acknowledge them as citizen.[41] Stateless persons may also be caught in the turmoil of war. In addition, in some cases, the state chooses at will to strip people of their citizenship. The Bengalis in Pakistan are neither refugees nor IDPs and, until 1971, were bona fide citizens of the country. They no longer enjoy that privilege.[42] Given the complexity of movement, rights, and citizenship, a person can simultaneously be a stateless person and a refugee.

Unfortunately, for a variety of reasons, the challenges of internally displaced and stateless communities, particularly in the Global South, are not nearly as well studied as those of refugees. This is not to say that the discipline of refugee studies does not suffer from bias or colonialism, which indeed has been well documented. It is to argue that the disciplines dealing with complex issues of internal displacement and statelessness are even more in need of research, scholarship, and local engagement. The reasons include limited interest from governments (many of which are complicit in creating the crises in the first place) to allow the access needed for research and scholarship.

IDPs, while distinct in many ways from those who cross international borders, may face many challenges similar to those faced by refugees.[43] These communities may not only be forced to live in "camps" or "settlements" for extended periods,[44] and their movement may be aggressively controlled, they may also face xenophobia, persecution, gender-based violence, and exclusion from public services in health, education, and employment.[45] Their long-term health indicators remain well-behind nondisplaced citizens.[46]

| Another inaccurate perception that is perpetuated by a uniform image of forcibly displaced persons is that they largely reside in refugee camps. While forced migration is not a recent phenomenon, the camp, as we imagine it, is not very old. Historians believe that the "camp" emerged in late nineteenth-century Ottoman era and became a common sight during the Armenian genocide crisis that led to the mass movement of Armenians from the Ottoman Empire to Syria and Lebanon.[47] Over the years, the organization, architecture, and control of the refugee camp also became a means of controlling lives, both for colonial power and for domestic political purposes.[48] Whether people were allowed to

leave and integrate depended on, among other things, the ethnicity, religion, and political and strategic interests of the colonial power.[49] Yet, despite the presence of camps in nearly all countries that have refugees (or perhaps precisely *because of* the characteristics of those camps), the majority of refugees do not live in these camps.[50]

In Pakistan, where Afghan refugees started to flee to in the late 1970s (by the end of 1980 there were more than four million Afghan refugees) and where today there are more than 1.4 million *registered* Afghan refugees, only a third of them live in refugee villages (*villages* is the term for camps in Pakistan),[51] while two-thirds of Afghan refugees live in urban areas.[52] Globally the percentage of refugees living in urban areas is about the same or even higher. UNHCR estimates suggest that nearly 75 percent of refugees *do not* live in camps.[53] Some refugees start out in camps, but as the crisis extends into an indefinite future and as camps become permanent, they leave for urban areas.[54] The reasons why refugees leave refugee camps are complex[55] and range from limited economic opportunity offered in the camps, to family ties in the urban centers, to anxiety about the colonial nature and excessive control of life in the camp, to increased and immediate access to health care outside the camps. In the case of refugees or migrants who are unregistered, or do not wish to register, urban areas offer anonymity, which the camps do not.[56] Life outside the camps also offers a connection to the social network that provides protection, information, and economic opportunity.[57] Similar reasons drive movement of IDPs from camps to urban or peri-urban areas. In Yemen, for example, several communities have had to move from one city to a camp, to another camp, and then to another city, as the conflict escalates.[58]

Variety of Camps

Unlike the pictures that may appear in newspapers or in promotional materials from NGOs, camps, like the people living in them, are not uniform.[59] Not only do they vary in size, each camp is a mixture of a formal structure (imposed by an outside agency) and an organic structure, which evolves from within and changes with time.[60] Health care access and services, for example, are complex and often lack a single cohesive structure.[61] There may be a formal health unit in the camp with a pharmacy, and yet there may be, located near it, informal stores that also serve as pharmacies.

Also lost in a uniform image of a refugee camp is the complexity of multiple ethnicities or nationalities living together. In central Beirut's Shatila camp, Palestinian refugees and Syrian refugees live side by side,[62] even though the Palestinians may have arrived decades before the Syrians. Uganda has South Sudanese refugees living in camps (of various sizes) as well as refugees from Congo, who make up 25 percent of its refugee population.[63] In Colombia, internally displaced persons live alongside Venezuelan refugees and indigenous people.[64] In urban slums of Karachi (there are no formal camps), there are stateless Bengali persons and internally displaced Pashtuns in the same neighborhoods.[65]

Conflicted Relationship with the State and Local Community

The picture of a refugee completely dependent on an international agency may make a good argument for fundraising, but the reality is not as straightforward. Those who are displaced (both refugees and IDPs) have a complex relationship with the state and even the local government.[66] While the term *host nation* is often used, it does not always indicate a willing or a gracious community that is welcoming toward those who come from outside. The reception of a local government to those from outside its region is influenced by local and national history, prior experience with refugees, the political atmosphere prevailing in the country, and interactions between the government and the international donor community.[67] The same community—for example, those displaced by the Syrian civil war—may be housed in large, organized camps in Jordan and Turkey and in informal settlements in Lebanon.[68] The Lebanese policy has a lot to do with Lebanon's fifteen-year civil war,[69] its experience with Palestinian refugees, and support for the Assad regime among powerful political and sectarian groups that have a strong influence on the Lebanese government.

Venezuelans forced to migrate due to the economic collapse of the nation found completely different policies for housing, health care, and integration in the three neighboring states of Brazil, Ecuador, and Colombia.[70] Despite a large number of refugees, there are countries, such as Colombia, where there are *no* formal camps.[71] In these places there may emerge, from time to time, neighborhoods (often lacking basic resources) where a higher number of refugees live, alongside locals and internally displaced persons.

Whether a country has formal camps or not, the presence of a large number of displaced populations results in a multidimensional relationship with the local host community. This relationship is distinct from the formal relationship with an aid agency or even with the national government. The relationships between the host community and the displaced community are often complex.[72] Those who are displaced often have personal and family relationships in the host community and often engage in transactions that affect access to food, employment, and health care.[73]

Causes of Displacement

Just as the housing situations for refugees vary, so do the reasons why people are forced to leave their homes. While war and armed conflict continues to drive a significant number of people toward safety, the economic collapse of a state is also a major reason for mass migration, both within the country (such as in Zimbabwe[74]) or across international borders (such as those leaving Venezuela). In some cases, economic collapse in a single country leads to both internal displacement and the crossing of international borders (e.g., some Zimbabwean migrants moved within their country and some moved to South Africa). Because economic collapse and subsequent migration was historically not used as a refugee classification, providing care and assistance has been challenging and inconsistent, especially in light of unclear international treaties and mandates.[75]

Refugee health—historically and in practice—has often been viewed through the lens of humanitarian emergencies, such as famine, natural disasters, and conflict.[76] As a result, there has been an oversized emphasis on immediate needs of food, water, immunization, and prevention and control of infectious diseases. Many international agencies support efforts to control extreme malnutrition and to deliver immunizations; indeed a significant number of physicians engaged in refugee work are infectious disease experts. This emphasis on "emergency" has meant that health care challenges emerging from protracted crises are poorly understood and not given adequate attention.[77] The number of mental health professionals, for example, are miniscule despite growing evidence of the severity of mental health crises among forcibly displaced communities.[78] The health care of stateless communities remains largely ignored and mired in legal complexities.[79] On the ground, the situation mirrors the absence of scholarship. Issues of trauma and mental health, likely stemming from exclusion, xenophobia, stress, and lack of basic attention, are rarely addressed. In Karachi's Machar Colony there is only one mental health clinic for a community of several hundred thousand.

Long-term Needs of Displaced Persons

In dealing with emerging and existing health challenges among refugees and IDPs, one troubling approach is to rigidly separate how infectious diseases versus chronic ailments are addressed. This separation has resulted in chronic diseases (e.g., diabetes, cancer, mental health) getting less attention and funding than they deserve.[80] The separation also uses more resources than a more effective, integrated approach would use. The lack of interest and limited emphasis on strengthening the health system by taking a more holistic approach has worried experts regarding the impact of COVID-19 on displaced communities.[81] While early data suggests that the impact of COVID-19 on refugees worldwide has been relatively modest compared to some countries, the long-term impact remains a serious concern. It is possible that a relatively modest mortality rate comes from misreading existing data or from the lack of data collected to date.[82] Also, data about the pandemic's impact on refugees has come largely from camp populations and not from refugees living elsewhere or from IDPs; these groups have their own unique health challenges.[83] Furthermore, data is often self-reported by governments and therefore can be viewed with skepticism, especially data from places like Yemen, where there is a general denial about the pandemic's existence or lethality.[84] In places like South Sudan, data from rural areas, where displaced communities often reside, is nearly nonexistent.

Beyond the debate on mortality rates, there are longer-term aspects of the pandemic that continue to concern public health experts. In Yemen, where there are extraordinarily high levels of malnutrition, poor access to health care among displaced persons, and a cholera outbreak, COVID-19 will have serious consequences.[85] In Afghanistan, COVID-19 is one of several outbreaks simultaneously impacting health care;[86] the outbreaks include malaria, dengue, cholera, and measles. In addition, communities of displaced persons already experience high levels of hypertension and anxiety; therefore, separating the impact of the pandemic from mental health would create both short- and long-term problems, especially in communities who have been pushed or nudged to "return home" due to the pandemic (as in in Colombia[87] and Uganda).

Journeys Are Not Unidirectional

Finally, the image of refugees as persons on a journey that moves in one direction only is also inaccurate and dangerous. It is often assumed that refugees leave a country, move to another country, and continue on their journey until they settle (mostly in Western Europe, and in the United States). Or—in some cases—they repatriate to their home country. This is both historically and statistically inaccurate. Refugees might go back and forth between their home country and their transitional country several times,[88] sometimes by choice (e.g., to seek care, to attend to personal issues) and sometimes by force. This is risky, not only because of potential health and safety consequences but also because aid providers might consider leaving the camp an act of repatriating (based on inflexible bureaucratic models) and might change the status of the displaced person with international agencies. Yet, this happens routinely. Refugees may rely on complicated networks and means to evade authorities. There is also the issue of what "transient" and "permanent" means and how they are interpreted.[89] The created image fails to account for people who go back and forth repeatedly, or those who return home but are forced to flee again. Or those who are forced to flee their camp if their new country becomes unsafe, as was the case with Palestinian refugees who first moved to Syria, and then, after spending decades there, were forced to flee again due to the conflict that started in 2013.[90]

Just as movement to another country is often assumed to be temporary, repatriation itself can be temporary. Displaced communities may view borders completely differently[91] than researchers and distant observers. This impermanence is not only problematic when looking at composite statistics, but it also creates a restricted narrative, where help and support is provided only if someone is "displaced." But their situations are erased from international help and support if they "return" to their prior communities or come back "home" to communities lacking in basic services and security. This lack of attention and services forces people to move again.[92] A uniform image can make a situation full of harrowing statistics fit a particular, tidy narrative, but it's unlikely to honestly portray the lived experiences of displaced persons.

Chapter 2
A Brief History of Forcibly Displaced Persons and Refugee Camps

Rafael settles into his new life in Bogotá among other Venezuelan refugees

Rafael's room in the shared apartment in Bogotá was smaller than the smallest room in his house in Lecheria. It had off-white walls with chipping paint and a brown water stain in the middle of the ceiling. Rafael wondered if this was a stain from water leakage some time ago or if this was a sign that the roof might suddenly collapse on him. Despite the unnerving stain and the size of the room, he felt lucky. At least he had a roof over his head. And a bathroom, albeit shared, with running water.

He'd found the place through family. A distant relative on his mother's side had been living in Bogotá for some time. Rafael had reached out to her, through some friends on a borrowed phone, after he'd decided he would be going to Colombia and found out that she had a spare room in her apartment. It wasn't free, but it was available immediately to rent at a reasonable rate. He could also defer the first month's rent until he'd found work. The unwritten contract suited Rafael just fine.

Rafael had been to Bogotá before but had never been to this part of town. The jungle of apartments in this working-class neighborhood was something completely new to him. In his prior trips, he'd had no reason to come to this area. Last time he was in Bogotá, years ago, he was welcomed by the shopkeepers and the waiters at the restaurants because they knew he had money to spend. Not anymore. His Venezuelan accent had not been an issue last time. It was now. People's attitude changed when he spoke, and at the grocery store he felt the weight of the shopkeeper's stare on his back. Uncomfortable, frustrated, and anxious, Rafael went out less and less, or if he would go out, he wouldn't talk to anyone he didn't know. The one big exception was Venezuelans. He would talk to them endlessly. There were many of them here, including some from his hometown by the sea.

Venezuelans had been coming to Bogotá for decades to study, do business, party, and work. Some had married and settled. But now there were others like him, who had come unwillingly and more recently. Rafael—through his landlady—got to know many of them. These Venezuelans were not like the businessmen or lawyers like him who had visited before. There were no hotel accommodations for them anymore. These people lived in squalid conditions,[1] in apartments that were even more cramped than his.

Rafael met people from all types of backgrounds. He came across workers and farmers, doctors and nurses, retired accountants and teachers. He met a nurse from Venezuela who couldn't access medicine for her two children, both with severe asthma, for weeks until one's condition got so bad that he had to be admitted to the hospital in the emergency room. There was a professor who was trying to get his degree validated despite his thirty-seven years of experience teaching at a university in Venezuela. There was a pediatrician, a mother of two young children, who had traveled in a cramped bus for two nights, trying to evade the authorities as she entered Colombia illegally. When she reached the bridge in Cúcuta, it was raining so hard that the water was up to her knees. With her children in her arms, she felt that her legs would not be able to carry her across the bridge.

And then there was Olga, a seventy-two-year-old woman and a poet, who had worked all her life in Paraguaná Peninsula, in western Venezuela. As the economic crisis intensified, she saw her city and the society crumble around her. People that she had known all her life were leaving her city one by one. She knew she'd have to leave as well, but she kept delaying for as long as she could. And then one day Olga's best friend, Alicia, got sick and the hospital could not take care of her. There were few doctors—most had left the country—and even fewer medicines. Alicia's illness was treatable, but she died. Her death left a permanent hole inside Olga. On the day of her death, Olga knew it was time to go.

When Olga arrived home from the hospital, she instinctively started cleaning the place as if she would never return. She wanted to leave her home in pristine condition for whoever would be the new occupant. Her house was beautiful and had a big parlor and high ceilings. She'd lived there all her life; it was the place that connected her to her parents. The thought of leaving the most peaceful place in her life was heartbreaking. She dusted the paintings and arranged the chairs around the dining table. She wiped the counters and scrubbed the toilet. Then she took out just enough clothes that could fit in a backpack. She swung the backpack on her shoulder and left, without looking back.

She took a bus to San Cristobal, sitting alone for the entirety of the long trip. From San Cristobal, she took a taxi to Cúcuta and waited at the border while the guards checked passports. Much to her surprise, the border crossing was uneventful. Maybe her age gave her immunity from the excessive questioning that she'd heard about from other people. After crossing the border, she waited for the bus to take her to Bogotá on a fifteen-hour journey.

Olga's bus kept stopping and breaking down. Anxious, alone, hungry, and tired, she finally reached Bogotá after several days. Initially, she found a place with some relatives who had been living in the city. They were kind to her, but Olga knew that they were struggling themselves and did not have the means to support her forever. She tried to look for a job, as a teacher, editor, bookkeeper, social worker, or even a waitress. No one wanted to hire a chronically ill seventy-two-year-old. Olga needed medications to manage her chronic pains, and she was told she was eligible for state care. Since she had entered the country legally, she had even gotten an insurance document (called Entidades Promotoras de Salud, or EPS) that said so. But appointments could only be made on the phone, and every time she called, no one picked up.

Rafael met many people like Olga, people who were trying to create new lives in a new place and trying to get food and medicine in a complicated and unfamiliar system. But not everyone Rafael met had a degree, had worked at a university, or was interested in the arts. There were old men and women, farmers and carpenters, drivers and grocers, families with young children. And then there were young girls. Teenagers working in the underbelly of Bogotá, forced into prostitution.[2] There was a demand and a supply of vulnerable girls. No one wanted to recognize this problem, which had spiraled out of control. Yet, everyone knew about it. These young girls needed social, psychological, and medical care. There were HIV cases and an increase in sexually transmitted diseases.[3] There were pregnancies and abortions, infections and trauma.

Rafael was the only lawyer among the Venezuelans he knew. Initially his law degree and his license to practice in Venezuela was of little practical use in Bogotá. The system in Colombia was different than what he'd been trained for. As a Venezuelan, with no local license, he could not practice in Bogotá. Through his family contacts and some new friends, Rafael had found work in an NGO that was providing assistance to Venezuelan refugees. This NGO worked with Venezuelans who needed medical and legal support for basic needs. The organization was supported by private donors from the United States and had infrequent support from the mayor's office in Bogotá.

Most of the Venezuelans Rafael interacted with were in need of some kind of medical care. Some had serious needs, like surgery; others needed regular attention, including those with AIDS or cancer. The system in Colombia was opaque and cumbersome. There was a lot of paperwork required to figure out who was entitled to what. The bureaucracy barely kept up with those who were in the country legally. For those who were under the radar and had arrived in the country illegally (whom Rafael worked with the most), the system simply did not work.

Technically Rafael was not working as a lawyer, but he liked to imagine that the Venezuelans who needed his help were somehow his responsibility. In Venezuela, Rafael had largely worked for organizations and companies—banks, housing societies, insurance companies—and individuals who were trying to protect their assets. He had never worked as a social worker. He knew little about hospitals, medicines, and the right to health care. In his prior life, Rafael could distance himself, and his life, from the institutions he represented. It was different now. Now he was part of the very same community, forcibly displaced from home and longing for family.

Henry prepares for Solomon's return

Henry was preparing for his brother Solomon's return from the refugee camp in Uganda. Henry—in an old Nissan 4 × 4 that he'd borrowed from a friend—drove from Malakan to Juba, the capital of South Sudan and his current home. Henry needed to bring supplies and furniture from his home in Malakan so he would be prepared for Solomon. On the map it was 130 kilometers, but it always took him at least four hours. He wanted to be as prepared as possible to greet his brother.

On both sides of the road, there were signs and billboards sponsored by aid agencies touting the generosity of various nations. The billboards, all white with clear black writing and a customary picture of smiling locals and the requisite European or US flags, reminded the people of South Sudan that Americans, Norwegians, Danes, Germans, British, and Japanese had helped provide the people of South Sudan clean water, wider roads, public parks, hospitals, dispensaries, and contraception.

The advertised benevolence of the kind people from the north was unmistakable. Unfortunately, none of the things advertised were evident as Henry drove on the unpaved dirt road. Despite the omnipresent signs and announcements, he was told by his friends that the number of signs here was just a fraction of the number in and around Bidi Bidi.

In the shadow of the billboards which had now rusted, there were, however, new dwellings appearing all over the region. Dwellings that weren't there just a few months ago. People like Solomon were coming back to South Sudan and trying to settle in the lands they'd left years ago. Henry had met some of these families in his church in Malakan. He couldn't tell whether they were excited to be back or not. Were they relieved? Were they satisfied with their decision? Henry was not sure. Some were genuinely happy to be back among family, but even the relieved ones seemed tired and exhausted. Some had left the camps because life had gotten too hard and too dangerous to navigate. Others were worried about COVID-19.

The dwellings that were going up in and around Malakan were mostly made of mud and local bush. The materials were provided by the church, local charities, and NGOs. Inside a boundary wall built with dried brush, there were two or three rooms that were not connected. The rectangular perimeter of the dwelling was marked by dried brush, tied together and erected upright. Some families that returned had started to cultivate the tiny plot of land next to the dwelling. Henry saw women tilling the land. Members of his church told him that they were starting to plant cassava and groundnuts with equipment they could borrow from friends, family, or the church. The equipment loan system, that had developed organically, seemed to be working for the families.

The new dwellings weren't located directly next to each other; there was barren land in between, used to store bush, stone, or trash. Plastic bottles and plastic bags, strewn in empty areas, were visible from a distance in a landscape that otherwise had no fluorescent colors.

Not all dwellings were made out of brush and thatched roofs. Occasionally Henry would pass by a house under construction with a brick and stone structure, tied together with sticky clay or, in some cases, cement. These homes also had a boundary wall. The metal beams sticking out of the incomplete walls present a jarring contrast to the other dwellings, which were constructed without any steel or metal. Henry knew that bricks were not cheap, so the occupants probably had relatives in Juba or abroad who helped them financially.

On one of his trips, as Henry was about to leave Malakan and get on the big road to Juba, he decided to take a detour. There was a place he needed to visit. So he turned around, drove to his one-room church, and parked. In the distance, next to the big tug tree, was a four-room building with a metal sheet roof. A new primary school was coming up. About two hundred yards from there was another building; it was painted light yellow with a red roof. This building was his destination.

"Good morning, Reverend," an elderly man said as Henry approached.

"How are you, Joseph?"

"Very fine, sir."

They chatted about Joseph's family and the primary school. There were no kids there today.

Next, Henry inquired about the place he'd visited many times. "Is there anyone there?"

"No. No one here."

The door was locked with a big gray lock, but Henry had the keys. It was the golden one in his set. He opened the door and immediately felt the waft of dust. It was dark. He knew exactly where the light switch was, and he flipped it. Nothing happened. No power, again. Henry peeked in. Everything looked the same. Nothing but layers of dust had come in since Henry had locked it two months ago. The room looked exactly the same, with tools that didn't work, a refrigerator plugged into a socket didn't have power, and cabinets that remained bare.

Making a mental note of the drugs that he would try to locate in Juba and bring with him on his next trip, Henry locked the door of the primary health facility and walked back to his car. There might be new people in town, Henry thought, but some things remained the same.

Saida becomes
head of her household

The colony's name, *Machar*, came from the Bangla word that meant fisherman, which reflected the history and the tradecraft of most Bengalis who lived in the slum. Over the years the word got distorted and people forgot what the original term was. The colony was not called *Machaira* (the Urdu word for fisherman) but called *Machar*, the Urdu word for a mosquito, a derogatory term. When someone from outside the colony heard the name, they sometimes chuckled. Even major newspapers report as if the origin of the name was related to the mosquito[4] without considering the Bangla origin of the word and its association with the residents' work. The racist undertone wasn't hard to miss. It suited the outsiders just fine and painted a perfect picture of the slum in their mind. The people in the colony were living in a filthy environment; they existed as a nuisance and needed to be squatted away. Or, if the outsiders happened to be benevolent and didn't want to get rid of the colony, the best thing they could do was to avoid the mosquitos. The name *Machar* was quite apt in their minds.

Saida didn't have time to worry about what the outsiders called her. She had more immediate needs, like being able to survive and have enough to eat. In the last two months, all she'd eaten was stale bread. Her brother, Tanvir, would show up at the nearby restaurant at night, after it had closed for the day, and collect pieces of bread. These were burnt, raw, or brittle, and these are what the family survived on. Saida had developed a method to make the bread edible. She'd carefully separate the burnt pieces from the ones that were cooked. She'd soak them in water, and then dry them just long enough that they were no longer soggy but before they became too brittle again. Saida knew that there was no nutrition in the meal, but it was enough to save them from starving.

By local social standards, Saida shouldn't have been at the bottom of the economic ladder in the community because there were two men at her home: Tanvir, who was in his thirties, and her son, who was seven. She was technically married as well, since her husband had never divorced her. He'd simply sent her back to her family but still retained all his rights over her and denied her any rights. Yet it was Saida who'd become the de facto head of the household. Her mother did have a say in day-to-day matters and was formally the head of the household, but she was getting old and not doing well.

It hadn't always been this bad. Saida got married when she was young and had lived with her husband for three years. She'd accepted her lot—an abusive husband who was also a drug addict. This was the norm in the community. Everyone Saida knew had been physically abused by their fathers, elder brothers, and husbands. Heroin and hashish were available on the street. In her eyes, she wasn't much worse than everyone else she knew. But what started as a norm, deteriorated quickly in her home. Things had come to a head five years ago, when her husband asked Tanvir for money. It was probably for his drug addiction, but he told Tanvir that he needed to start a business. Maybe the money was for both.

Tanvir didn't have any money, so he flatly refused.

Saida's husband had little patience for rejection, especially by his in-laws. In Machar Colony, as in many other parts of Pakistan, men like Saida's husband felt a tremendous sense of entitlement toward their in-laws. The fact that he was keeping Saida in his house, and providing for her, should have been enough for her family to accept all his demands. Saida's husband did not take kindly to this refusal. Initially, he swallowed his pride and waited to come back another day. A few weeks later, he returned. He knew Tanvir didn't have any money, so he asked Tanvir to sell his motorcycle. Tanvir refused. Saida's husband beat up Tanvir and came home. He verbally, and then physically, attacked Saida. He sent her back to her mother's home that same evening. She arrived physically bruised and emotionally distraught, with her infant son.

Tanvir, according to the norms and expectations of the colony, should have been the one looking after the family, but he was a vulnerable person. Tanvir and Saida's father, like Saida's husband, had been abusive and an addict. Years ago, he'd left the family to fend for itself. Saida and Tanvir grew up with their mother, as their father moved out, remarried, and erased his previous family from his life. He was still around, living in the colony, just not in their lives.

Despite limited means, Tanvir's mother sent him to school. Young Tanvir was a boy of small frame. He was bullied by other kids and sexually assaulted at the school by one particular teacher. The scars from the sexual abuse would remain in Tanvir's life and would shape the life of his whole family for decades.

Without a father, undernourished, and with no social support, Tanvir was an easy target for bullying and abuse. He had no real social network to support him and couldn't fight back. The abuse at the school continued. It eventually became too much for him; ultimately Tanvir dropped out of school. At home he was always anxious and scared. He stopped talking to anyone except his mother and his sister. Now that he was no longer in school, people in the colony suggested that he start earning money. But he wasn't getting any better. He developed severe depression (though it took years for it to be diagnosed), as he got caught up in a spiral of bad jobs, harassment, and low self-esteem. He was always in a disheveled state, with torn slippers and clothes with holes in them. He avoided eye contact, and people struggled to hear him when he spoke. In the cutthroat world of Machar Colony, where only the fittest had any chance of survival, some called him a curse on the family, others suggested using force to straighten him out. The neighbors swore by their methods of using chains to tie up people like Tanvir to get them back to being normal. But Saida and her mother resisted. They knew Tanvir wasn't a bad person or possessed by demons; nor was he under the spell of a jealous relative. He was sick and needed treatment. Few agreed, and their community left the family to live out its days in misery.

Tanvir, on the other hand, contemplated ending his own life. Twice he tried to commit suicide, but Saida had found out just in time and had intervened. Saida knew that while she'd been lucky two times, she might not get another chance. Though she'd never gone to school, she'd heard from others that there was help available for people like Tanvir.

She just had to find it.

A short history of global politics, refugee camps, and humanitarian organizations

"Camps seem to be everywhere and nowhere at the same time," Irit Katz notes.[5] The camp, in many ways, has not changed much in about a hundred years.[6] While the temporary camp today may consist of square or conical dwellings made out of prefab material, covered by blue or white tarp with a big emblem of the UNHCR or the International Organization of Migration (IOM)—things that were not there a hundred years ago—the overall organization of the camp has remarkable similarities to the first camps that appeared in towns in Iraq, Syria, and Lebanon in the 1920s and 1930s.[7] The camp today is often located at an optimal distance from the city: accessible but not too close. The equilibrium between control and social inconvenience has remained a stubborn hallmark of the camps.

Nearly a hundred years ago, and nearly three decades before the UNHCR was created (in 1950), new campsites were appearing in Europe (e.g., Greece) and the Middle East.[8] The shelters were made from thick, army-grade tent cloth, and the triangular architecture was supported not by walls but by a wooden pole. In many cases, the building material came directly from the colonial armies present in nearby countries.[9] In Baquba, Iraq, for example, the material came from the British army barracks in India.[10] The camp, as it emerged, was thought of as part of the solution, albeit a temporary one, to what was called "the refugee problem."[11] Those proposing the solution knew that it was temporary, but there was little agreement on what the permanent solution might look like. Discussions for that permanent solution—of integration and resettlement—in conferences all over Europe were affected by the milieu of regional and global politics, xenophobia, and pervasive racism.

Statelessness after the First World War

In the aftermath of the First World War, as old imperial structures crumbled, and new nation-states emerged in Europe and the Middle East, a new problem had emerged: the situation of statelessness.[12] While persecution of individual groups based on religion or ethnicity and their subsequent migration was nothing new, and while there had been plenty of recent episodes of large-scale persecution (e.g., the migration to Western Europe and the United States in the aftermath of Jewish pogroms and systemic persecution in Imperial Russia that had gone on for decades), the collapse of the Russian, Ottoman, and Austro-Hungarian empires and the rise of new nation-states resulted in large numbers of people who no longer belonged to any state. This problem of statelessness—people without a country—began to dominate international politics and the emerging global world order. With newspaper stories and accompanying vivid imagery of stranded, helpless people, there was public pressure that demanded a solution.[13] Russian journalist Ariadna Tyrkova-Williams wrote in 1921, "Never in the history of Europe has a political cataclysm torn such huge numbers of people from their mother country and from their homes."[14] In the same year, weeks before Christmas, the Save the Children Fund included in its newsletter a photograph of nine refugee children from Saratov Province, accompanied by a poem by pacifist writer Israel Zangwill titled "They Might Be Yours."[15]

Many among those displaced were citizens of the former Russian Empire who were caught up in the First World War.[16] Tsar Nicolas II of Russia had led his country to war, and millions were sent to the frontlines. Some had willingly signed up; others were conscripted. The war didn't go well for Russia, a country that had already been struggling with repeated famines and a widening gap between the rich and poor, as well as increasing anger and frustration among the peasants and industry workers about food shortages, lack of political representation, and declining quality of life. The tsar's government limped on until 1917, and on March 15, with his abdication, the Romanov dynasty ended. The fall of Tsarist Russia, and the subsequent rise of Bolsheviks (led by Vladimir Lenin) who campaigned to end the war, created a new and unpredictable situation for those engaged at the battlefronts far from St. Petersburg. The Bolsheviks, on their end, were suspicious of former supporters and sympathizers of the tsar, many who were now far from home on the frontlines or prisoners of war all over Europe. The Bolsheviks worried that these battle-hardened soldiers, upon their return, could undermine the already fragile October Revolution. The fate of these Russian refugees now hung in the balance, and the post-war European and US leadership wanted a solution for these stateless people.[17]

Russians weren't the only ones who had become stateless. There were others, including Armenians facing a genocide carried out by the Ottoman government. As the First World War unfolded and Turkey faced invading armies on the eastern front, the government became concerned that many Armenians would defect to the Russian army. The government's response was to disarm their Armenian soldiers and simultaneously incarcerate, deport (at a short notice, with no provisions of food and water), and even deliberately kill Armenians living in Anatolia. Estimates of those killed varies from 300,000 to 1.5 million.[18] The deportation also led to the mass migration of nearly a quarter million Armenians, who went to Iran, Syria, Palestine, Jordan, Lebanon, and Egypt. To this day, the Armenian genocide has been denied by every successive Turkish government, regardless of its political ideology.[19]

By the end of the war, statelessness had become a much bigger issue than what individual humanitarian organizations, relying almost exclusively on private support, could solve. It was no longer about food, famine, or a natural disaster in a far-off land. There was also not much appetite among the triumphant European nations to settle these people in Western Europe and the United States. The sheer number of people without a state required treaties, contracts, and assurances that were only possible at the governmental level. This needed diplomacy at a new scale.

The recently formed League of Nations, created in 1920 in the aftermath of the First World War,[20] was an obvious choice for addressing the problem.[21] At the core of the issue was the notion of *citizenship* and *belonging*, and of *identity papers* to prove the relationship between a citizen and a state. In the absence of documents, there was no possibility of movement, labor, or eventual resettlement.

Fridtjof Nansen: Diplomat and Humanitarian

The man at the center of the effort to address the problem of Russian refugees was an explorer from a country far from the epicenter of the migration crisis: a Norwegian named Fridtjof Nansen.[22] Born in 1861 in Christiania (modern day Oslo), Nansen grew up near the forests, and exploring them became his favorite childhood pastime. He started to ski at age two and became known among his family for his daring adventures (including a ski jump attempt at age ten that nearly ended his life). After an unremarkable performance in high school, he enrolled at the university to study zoology. It was here that he had the opportunity to explore the Arctic on a trip recommended by his zoology professor. This trip, according to Nansen, led him "astray from the quiet life of science."[23] Nansen did eventually return to research but not in the same department. He became part of a neurology research team at the Bergen Museum, a university museum in Norway, and worked on projects that challenged existing notions, creating a whole new explanation of how the nervous system works. His heart, however, was never in the lab. He wanted to explore uncharted territories in ways that were considered too risky or simply impossible. Nansen was known for his ascetic lifestyle, self-belief, innovation, and ability to dream. These characteristics would serve him well, in the variety of careers he undertook in his life.

His first big adventure was in 1888 when he traversed Greenland on rudimentary cross-country skis. Nansen's skill in navigating unforgiving terrain proved that he could do what others thought was barely possible. His biggest accomplishment, however, was to go where no person had gone before: the North Pole.[24]

Nansen made a daring, three-year attempt to reach the pole, starting in 1893. He came closer than any human had before, getting to latitude 86 degrees and 14 minutes,[25] remarkably close to the North Pole (the exact position of the North Pole is at latitude 90 degrees from the equator; one latitude equals sixty minutes). The expedition came to be known as the *Fram* (meaning "forward") expedition, named after Nansen's ship. Nansen's autobiographical story of travel and survival, *Farthest North*, became a bestseller and remains popular among explorers and adventurers.

After the North Pole adventure, Nansen felt that his exploration days were behind him. He returned to the academy and became a professor in Oslo. But just when his previous explorer career was ending, a new one in international politics and diplomacy was beginning. Riding on his fame and respect among the public, Nansen spoke passionately about ending Norway's union with Sweden, and was soon chosen to be an ambassador of his newly independent nation to Great Britain.[26] While not quite a household name across the world, he was widely respected and admired in the European academic and political circles. He was an environmentalist, well before the term was used or associated with a conservation movement. He was also a humanitarian, troubled deeply by global conflict, especially the First World War.[27] He wrote passionately about the evil of war, calling it "the greatest confession of defeat of humanity, a degradation, devoid of meaning, an orgy of self-destruction in which nothing flourished by the lust for power, hatred and stupidity—the bitter fruits of which mankind must eat for a generation."[28]

Nansen, through his advocacy and political positions, found many admirers across the world, including in some unusual quarters. Peter Kropotkin, an ardent anarchist, considered him a hero.[29] In October 1923, *New York Times* journalist Hannah Astrup Larsen, a

Norwegian-American, wrote gushingly about Nansen, "The tall, commanding figure, the strong jaw, the dome-like forehead which seemed to bear down with its own weight, the fine wrinkles coming to a focus in the bright, scintillating eyes—the eyes of a sailor looking out over a sunny sea—all contributed to a look of austerity, which, however, soon resolved itself into intensity and concentration."[30]

In 1920, the League of Nations appointed Nansen as the first High Commissioner for the Prisoners of War with a goal of repatriating those interned in Russia, Germany, and regions of the former Austro-Hungarian Empire. Nansen's original mission was narrowly defined. This mission soon morphed into his position as High Commissioner for Russian Refugees and included stateless persons who may not have been prisoners. This new organization based in Geneva had extremely limited financial resources. On average, it was provided approximately 250,000 Swiss Francs per year. The resources for staff were even more modest. The staff consisted of a handful of people, handpicked by Nansen himself.[31]

While the narrow mandate was somewhat clear, the legal and juridical problems were quite the opposite. International law at the time stipulated that foreigners were subject to the laws of their own nations. For Russians stripped of their citizenship (or not granted any new citizenship by the Bolshevik government or any other country), the precarious situation of statelessness meant that basic issues of inheritance, marriage, divorce, and so on, could not be settled in any court. Nansen communicated with legal scholars (including Russian exiles) across Europe to figure out what to do. The scholars debated and then proposed new theoretical concepts and legal frameworks. But little headway was made for immediate action on the ground for those who urgently needed help. The easiest thing and one that found support in most legal and intellectual circles, as well as among major power brokers of the League of Nations, was repatriation: send people back to where they came from.[32]

The idea of repatriation was not in line with the major global political tides of the time, which focused on internationalism, a policy of cooperation among nations. Despite the intellectual attractiveness of internationalism and some progressive support for the idea in theory (including among prominent Soviet intellectuals[33]), the view that ultimately prevailed was a more conservative one that said, "A man was comfortable among his own people, on his own territory and that his return should be facilitated by all available means."[34]

The practical realities of sending people back to their "home," however, were significantly different from theoretical concepts about comfort and belonging among one's own people. While early efforts at repatriation seemed promising, the idea broke down quickly as Russia grappled with a severe famine and a civil war between the Reds (Bolsheviks) and Whites (supporters of the deposed tsar) in the new Soviet Union.[35]

There was also another, and perhaps fatal, flaw in the repatriation strategy. Those who had become stateless were largely members of communities that had fought against the Red forces in the civil war (that started soon after the Bolsheviks came to power), and their repatriation was likely to result in intense persecution by the Bolshevik authorities eager to exert their control and authority.[36]

Despite these warnings, repatriation was tried for a few months. Only a small number of people, roughly a few thousand, were sent back to their communities, as most Russian refugees remained skeptical of the Bolsheviks. In 1922, after two months of repatriations of Russian refugees from Bulgaria, the situation changed. Rumors of mass killings of repatriated Russians started to appear in Russian-language émigré newspapers.[37] This was deeply concerning for Nansen and his mission. His office tried but failed to get any reliable information about the well-being, or even the whereabouts, of those who had been sent back. Unconfirmed reports of ill treatment of repatriated Russians continued to trickle in for a few months. The problem was made even more complicated by a devastating famine in Russia and Ukraine, and a fact-finding mission could not be sent. Ultimately Nansen's team, as well as exiles from Russia, understood that repatriation was untenable as a policy to solve the problem of stateless Russians.[38]

Nansen had to change his approach.

The Nansen Passport

A lifelong innovator in all his pursuits, Nansen wasn't afraid to push the boundaries of what was considered possible. He and his office put forward a new, simple idea: allow people to move and settle temporarily, without formal citizenship papers, in a country that accepted refugees. Nansen's office, in partnership with the League of Nations, was going to provide a document that would be a substitute for formal identity papers for the stateless Russians who had none. This new idea first came to be known as the Nansen certificate, and eventually as the Nansen passport.[39]

The passport, first introduced in 1922, allowed holders to move to, and find work in, countries that would accept the document. Initially, twenty-four countries accepted the legality of the passport.[40] By 1942, fifty-two countries accepted it.[41] At first, only Russian refugees were issued the passport, but in 1924 the privileges were extended to Armenians, and in 1928 to Assyro-Chaldeans.[42] However, accepting a Nansen passport was not binding on any government, and the passport was not a universally accepted idea, particularly in some East European countries.[43]

The passport, while an innovative strategy and considered one of Nansen's signature achievements, offered little in terms of rights beyond the ability to move. Passport holders did not have a right to live permanently in a particular country. The passport was valid for only one year for most people, and for two years for Polish refugees.[44] Countries could send passport holders to adjoining countries, or they could expel them. The passports provided no path to naturalization and citizenship and no fundamental right to housing or access to health care. In case of outbreaks of diseases, which were increasingly frequent, the countries where refugees arrived were under no obligation to provide relief or grant access to health care facilities (if they existed). As the refugees faced epidemics of life-threatening infections, particularly typhoid and cholera, the burden of providing care fell on international humanitarian agencies, including the Red Cross, Save the Children, and Near East Relief.[45] These agencies worked closely with the League of Nations and contributed to the intellectual development of epidemic prevention and treatment, but their finances and leadership were independent of the League of Nations. Aid agencies depended on financial support from donors, philanthropists, and ordinary citizens to buy food in the case of famine, and to buy medicines and vaccines and to create quarantine centers, in the case of infectious diseases.[46]

The right of movement and labor and the right to access health care were dealt with separately from what the passport offered. In the immediate aftermath of the war, there was famine in Russia and repeated outbreaks of typhoid, syphilis, measles, and dysentery in several countries in Eastern Europe.[47] Refugees, and migrants already weakened by the war, were perfect hosts for pathogens. The influenza pandemic of 1918–1919, combined with ongoing typhoid epidemics, was particularly devastating for the forcibly displaced.[48] The pandemic also spread as the refugees and war prisoners migrated.[49] The Red Cross—both through its country offices and through partnership with other agencies—did its best to provide food and medical assistance, though its own internal politics and international diplomacy often got in the way of an effective response.[50]

The High Commissioner for Refugees continued to operate in the interwar period with a limited budget and a narrow mandate. But financial concerns were not the only challenge to its mission and mandate. It was facing new threats from the changing face of politics within several richer countries. The National Origins Act (1924) in the United States[51] and similar laws in Western Europe and Australia were passed to maintain a certain ethnic (i.e., white) composition of their population.[52] The rise of xenophobia, anti-Semitism, and racial prejudice resulted in countries closing their borders to immigrants from Asia.[53] With repatriation or resettlement in Europe and the United States becoming increasingly difficult, and with a continual increase in the number of people who needed to be protected, the vacuum was filled by the emergence of temporary shelters or camps, among other things.

The Camp as an Institution

Some of the early camps—present in Aleppo, Syria, and around Beirut (in modern-day Lebanon)—were initially run by humanitarian agencies and American and French missionaries.[54] Many of the workers had no language expertise, had no familiarity with the culture, or had not even traveled abroad previously. Now these people from the United States and Europe were making major decisions about food, water, shelter, and health care for millions of vulnerable people in a new land.

In time, the same camps were either run entirely by colonial powers or by partnerships between colonial authorities and missionary groups.[55] The efforts toward health care and humanitarianism also suffered from a colonial worldview of racism and exclusion where local populations were viewed as uncivilized or unhygienic. Institutions that focused on children and children's health prioritized children in Europe over those in the Middle East or South Asia. The focus on Europeans' well-being was so prominent that the first Save the Children Fund[56] meeting on improving the lives of non-European children didn't happen until 1931, despite the organization being in operation for well over a decade.[57] While multiple partners helped craft the policy, which ranged from food provisions to diplomacy, the camp emerged as a new fixture to regulate the lives of the poorest and weakest of the forced migrants.

The camp, as an institution, allowed for greater control over the lives of those within it. This, to a certain extent, is still true today.[58] In many instances the desire of the colonial powers in controlling the population's movement was central to the idea of the camp. In 1936 the French High Commissioner for Syria spoke about the French approach to the camps: "With the Armenians, what one fears is that as soon as they have a little savings, they will wish to go elsewhere. This must be avoided."[59] In other instances, colonial powers used the camps to enlist troops for specific missions that terrorized the local communities.[60]

Over the years, the camps became cities unto themselves and provided a clearinghouse and a valve to control immigration to Europe and the United States. With the rise of fascism and the Nazis in Italy and Germany, respectively, there was a concern about the rising number of European Jews who needed to be settled elsewhere. This realization led to conferences and discussions, most notably in Évian, France in 1938,[61] to come up with viable and permanent solutions. Those discussions were inconclusive. President Franklin Roosevelt wanted "the possibility of uninhabited or sparsely inhabited good agricultural lands to which Jewish colonies might be sent."[62] The problem for the Allied powers did not disappear even after the defeat of Germany. In the aftermath of the Second World War, those liberated from the Nazi-controlled concentration camps were housed in new refugee camps all over Europe, most notably in Germany, Austria, and Italy. Camps, in certain cases, were repurposed from Nazi concentration camps, with barbed wires and tight control on movement.[63] The former guard houses helped control populations within the camps.[64]

The problem was not just in Europe. In the post-war years, with the displacement of nearly three-quarter million Palestinians, new camps emerged in Jordan, Egypt, Syria, and Lebanon. The problem was so big that it required an entirely new agency, called the United Nations Relief and Works Agency (UNRWA), created in 1949.[65] That agency continues to operate today with an explicit mandate for the well-being of displaced Palestinians, including their health and education.[66] The management of UNRWA camps has not been without political interference, however. Historically, the United States had been the major financial supporter of UNRWA of its large programs focused on access to health care and education.[67] With changing political tides and increased nationalism in both the United States and Israel, this has started to change. The US support, previously considered a strategic investment, was abruptly stopped under the Trump administration and was hailed as a watershed moment, long overdue, by the (then) Netanyahu government in Israel.[68]

After the Second World War, new international structures for diplomacy and international governance emerged, most notably in the form of the United Nations. The world order had also changed, with the United States having a far greater say in diplomacy and international negotiations than in previous years. The Soviet Union's position was also cemented by its strong influence on the policy of a number of East European states. In the period between the end of the Second World War (1945) and the Refugee Convention (1951), where discussions were held about the definition of a refugee and the mandate of UNHCR, several new international organizational structures emerged. These included UNRRA (UN Relief and Rehabilitation Administration) and IRO (International Refugee Organization). Yet, despite the global mandate, these new structures maintained a colonial perspective, focusing largely on Europe and the Middle East. Their lack of interest in addressing problems that were not immediately threatening, or affecting, European and US political or financial interests significantly impacted refugee relief efforts in other parts of the world.[69]

Refugee Camps in India

In August 1947, British colonial governance of India ended, and what emerged was two new sovereign nations, Pakistan and India.[70] Border disputes, ethnic and communal clashes, and anxiety about the future led to one of the greatest episodes of mass migration.[71] While exact numbers are not available, it is estimated that nearly fifteen million people moved between India and Pakistan.[72] The violence preceding and accompanying the migration left traumatic scars. Those who arrived in the new lands often had little to support themselves. They were housed in makeshift camps that appeared in border cities.[73] Lahore, an ancient city in the newly created Pakistan, was home to several camps containing many people who were traumatized, injured, or sick. Old military barracks used by the Allied forces were repurposed to serve as refugee camps.[74] However, with as many as fifty thousand people crossing the border on some days, the camps were incapable of providing any real relief or shelter.[75] Families often camped by the roadside. With heavy rains in the monsoon season, and with extreme cold in the winter months, hundreds would die every day. This was in addition to the outbreaks of epidemics. Typhoid, diarrhea, and cholera outbreaks became routine, leading to a situation that reminded one aid worker of Dante's Hell. Dead bodies left by the roadside were collected daily for communal burials.

There was little help available to the new states in managing the humanitarian crisis. Despite visits by high-level government officials, UNRRA and IRO did not provide significant medical assistance to the displaced millions.[76]

The camps in Pakistan present a useful example of the chaos and of the woefully inadequate care provided by the main stakeholders.[77] The state was largely dysfunctional, in need of cash and in-kind support, and not interested in hosting refugees from India, despite its initial claim that Pakistan would be a home for all Muslims of India. Continued rioting on both sides of the border made migration along religious lines (Muslims from India to Pakistan, and Hindus and Sikhs from Pakistan to India) a mode of survival. The roads connecting the two new countries were often choked by people trying to migrate. The new refugees were often supported by local families, volunteers, international church-based charities, and global relief agencies like the Red Cross[78] but not by the state. Repeated outbreaks of typhoid, diarrhea, and cholera meant that the refugees needed both medical support and food assistance, but there was little from agencies headquartered in the West. Few doctors and volunteers with medical training were available.[79] Newspapers ran daily ads for donations of cash, blankets, and medical supplies. Inside the camps, the refugees were angry and frustrated and felt mistreated by the government authorities. There were riots, protests, and hunger strikes. The government responded by deploying armed police to maintain order. At the first anniversary of independence, the police fired on angry crowds and killed at least seventeen refugees.[80] Refugees who were sent from one province (Punjab) to the other (Sindh) for resettlement were beaten up and put back on the train. The government also maintained a strict censorship policy regarding news stories about the camps, and even fiction written during and about the period came under heavy scrutiny.[81]

Within a few years, the tented settlements of Lahore disappeared, and the population of poor refugees got absorbed or settled into local poverty (though ethnic fissures have remained). Today, it is almost impossible to find any trace of those camps, except in oral histories of the survivors and volunteers, or their descendants.[82]

But the disappearance of camps in low-income countries wasn't the norm. The Palestinian camps still exist, accommodating generation after generation. Even in Pakistan, the camps created for Afghan refugees—who arrived in large numbers in late 1970s—still endure.[83] Camps in Kenya (Dadaab) and Uganda (Bidi Bidi) have continued to grow over the decades and shelter several generations of families, including children born in the camps. Today, camp size varies from location to location, but those camps that survive beyond a few years tend to grow over time and often develop their own organic economic structure, connecting the local population, government, international agencies, and inhabitants of the camp. These complex structures have their own hierarchy and rules[84] that regulate nearly all facets of daily life, including access to resources and services.[85]

Current Camps

Today, camps might be referred to in more palatable terms, such as *tented* or *informal settlements* or *refugee villages*,[86] yet they all convey a similar meaning. They all are refugee camps. A camp remains a high-density environment, housing refugees who are among the poorest and most dispossessed of migrants. It is a place run by an international agency (typically UNHCR or IOM), in partnership with the local government. These camps are largely present in low- and middle-income countries. There are other off-shore models, such as the Australian asylum detention centers in Papua New Guinea and Nauru, which have been universally condemned for their inhumane conditions.[87]

Despite the variation in size, the camp architecture, at a higher level, is designed to convey particular messages: control and impermanence.[88] Dwellings are made from only a few types of materials, though there are several other materials that may be more cost effective and humane.[89] Yet, the refugees often have no access (either due to cost or restrictions) to materials to build their dwellings, and they are provided with specific materials to build their tents. There is also a strong resistance to changing the architecture, lest it give any indication of permanency. Even with prefabricated materials, the image is of something put up overnight, during an unpredictable emergency, and of something that could be dismantled in a similarly short period. The Syrian camps in Lebanon are a clear example: brick-and-mortar structures, even rudimentary ones, are specifically forbidden by the government.[90]

Refugees who are aware of the control the camp and local authorities want to enforce on their lives often choose to live outside the camps. The decision is not driven by a single reason, rather it is a product of several interlinking factors.[91] These include increased surveillance, poor treatment by the authorities, fear of living under a microscope, lack of economic opportunity and educational facilities, poor access to health care, and distrust of the local government despite their claims of job opportunities and special economic zones.[92] Those who choose to live in urban environments are often forced to live in urban slums or in shanties that suffer from poverty and neglect.[93] With limited sanitation and public services, these environments not only trap communities in a vicious poverty cycle but also create a near continuous exposure to infectious diseases.

Repatriation

As it was in Nansen's time, repatriation remains a preferred option of international agencies, and repatriation scores political points for the host communities as well, but the challenges facing those who return to their home country are also eerily similar to the ones faced by stateless

Russian refugees who were encouraged to go back to Russia nearly a hundred years ago. Concerns about safety and security, upon repatriation, are not insignificant. The Rohingya in Bangladesh and the Syrians in the Middle East and Europe are reluctant to return, just as the stateless Russian refugees were reluctant to return.[94] But there's more. The refugees who return (willingly or under coercion) and are not in a danger of state-sponsored persecution are greeted with a near complete absence of support services, destroyed as a result of conflict or economic collapse.[95] It is unclear who is responsible for the health and well-being of those who return. Since they may be transient, should they continue to be under the UNHCR mandate or does their well-being become the responsibility of the state? The returnees, such as South Sudanese who return from Uganda, may come under the mandate of a different international agency because in their own country they are no longer refugees, technically speaking.[96] The handover from one agency to another is anything but smooth and leaves many to fall through the cracks.

Those who do come back and attempt to rebuild their lives in a land that was once familiar, find rebuilding to be a complicated process, dependent for basic provisions on available resources, social networks (new and previous), and the presence of international agencies. In places like South Sudan, particularly in rural areas, there is a complete absence of services. The land, which may have been cultivable some time ago, may now be damaged due to conflict. Building supplies are often scarce and have to be shared among many. Schools and clinics may not be available, or if they are, they may remain understocked and with no trained staff.[97] Among those who do make the journey back, some choose to return to the refugee camp,[98] where they often have to re-register for the limited services.

Camps for internally displaces persons (IDPs), like those in Yemen, are supported by a consortium of agencies including the UNHCR and IOM.[99] The communities living in these camps are not technically refugees, yet their experiences are similar to the experiences of refugees. The material with which the camp housing is built seems like standard fare, produced en masse with big, bold emblems of international agencies.[100] While the IDP camps may not be UNHCR camps per se, the architecture, environment, and access to water, food, and medical services has strong similarities to refugee camps. It is the camp and its structure, and not the citizenship of residents, that often dictates health outcomes. The IDPs have health outcomes that are significantly poorer than health outcomes of nondisplaced citizens and that might even be worse than the outcomes of refugees.[101] The camp residents in IDP camps face similar challenges of insecurity as refugees. Lack of proper sanitation means that sewage gets mixed with drinking water, creating epidemics of diseases like cholera.[102]

For treatment, these communities are dependent for support on the outside (i.e., outside the camp, and often outside the country). Medical services are provided in the form of mobile health teams[103] that come from the city but that are dependent on the security situation. The services themselves (personnel, diagnostics, and medicines) are often dependent on international aid, and as that aid dries up or is delayed due to security issues, the health care offered to IDPs suffers drastically.[104] There are often long gaps between visits by the mobile health teams, yet there is little help available within the camps. In the absence of formal pharmacies, or with pharmacies that may charge significant fees, the vacuum in the camp is filled by unregulated pharmacies and medicines sold without a prescription.[105] It is no surprise, given this ad hoc system, that IDPs, like refugees, prefer to live in the city and not in the camp.[106] Many, however, are forced to live in camps due to economic, social, and political circumstances.

The camp model—tried, tweaked, and tested for nearly a century—is going strong. Yet no one, not even UNHCR, despite running hundreds of camps around the world, thinks it is the right solution for refugees or IDPs. In a policy announced in 2014, UNHCR said, "Camps should be the exception and, to the [furthest] extent possible, a temporary measure."[107]

In reality, they are the default and anything but the exception.

Chapter 3
Models of Health Care Systems

Rafael gets a job helping refugees access health care

After a month in Bogotá, Rafael had a regular routine for his days. He would wake up around seven o'clock in the morning and eat a small breakfast. While eating, he would read the news from back home in an attempt to maintain some semblance of a normal life, like the one that he'd had in Venezuela. But unlike in Lecheria, there was no newspaper here on his table. He read the news on his phone. And what he read was from a patchwork of places: actual news organizations, blogs, videos, and forwarded WhatsApp messages. Most of what was happening in Venezuela was predictable, but it was still discomforting. Political anxiety and propaganda at the national level, crime and hunger at the local level. WhatsApp messages were more specific, and more personal, but not always accurate. Rafael had learned how to mentally filter what (he thought) was fact from what (he perceived) was not, but the WhatsApp messages gave him a sense of what others were thinking and sharing.

Overall, what he was reading was not encouraging, and he often wondered if he could ever go back.

Occasionally Rafael also read the Colombian news, but for some reason this was even more discouraging. He had higher expectations of Colombia than he had of Venezuela, and he was worried that Colombia was becoming a pre-Chávez Venezuela, where a strongman could appear, promise everyone the moon and more, and take over the government as an authoritarian leader. Reading about a collapsed state was somehow easier for Rafael than reading about one at risk of collapsing.

In addition, his breakfast was a far cry from what he used to eat. Each morning he had only a cup of black coffee and a piece of bread. Despite all the things he no longer had, he liked having a routine.

After breakfast, Rafael would check up on his daughters. Mostly, he texted them because both the Wi-Fi connection in his room and their connection in Venezuela were weak and unreliable. Calls were hard because the connection was unstable, and both Rafael and his daughters would get frustrated. After initially trying to make it work for weeks, both sides decided that text was a better option.

Early morning texting with his daughters was his fuel to get through the day. He needed assurance that his daughters were fine, and that nothing had happened to them since he'd last heard from them. He mostly discussed how they were doing, and he wanted to sound positive. Conversations were more about them than about him. It wasn't that he had nothing to share, quite the contrary, but he was conflicted about what to say and how much to tell his daughters. On one hand, he didn't want to tell stories of life around him, about people and their struggles. That would be too hard on his daughters and make them worried about his own safety and well-being. The sad stories would demoralize his daughters even more. But, on the other hand, he knew his daughters had their own struggles living in Venezuela, and he wanted them to know he hadn't abandoned them. He didn't want them to think that he was now enjoying a better life than them, all by himself. The easiest thing was to talk mostly about them and less about him and his work.

His daughters would tell him about what happened the day before and who was doing what. There were stories about neighbors and boys, about their mother and relatives, just like the conversations they'd had before Rafael left the country. His daughters would also tell Rafael about what was going on at school. Despite everything that was going on, the schools were still open, even when many children had left the cities or the country altogether. Rafael was in awe of the teachers: they were not only a source of education but also a source of mental well-being in a society where so much was going wrong. And for many students, the schools were also a source of food, a daily meal for those who had little available at home. Though this was becoming less frequent, and some schools had stopped providing meals altogether.[1] Rafael often wondered how long the teachers would continue to teach before it became impossible. Some teachers, his daughters had told him, had already packed up and left.

On days when there was a Wi-Fi problem, or his daughters didn't write back, he felt tired, edgy, and incapable of concentration. Lately, things had been okay, given everything that was happening. His daughters were fine, almost chirpy. Even their mother, whom the girls were living with and whom Rafael did not talk to very often, had communicated with him to tell him that the girls were fine.

One day, Rafael opened his email as usual. This was a Monday, the day of the week that he received the most messages because it included the weekend's mail. The messages started to download slowly. Typically, he received email from two kinds of people: people newly arrived in Colombia who wanted access to health care and people who had already tried but were denied the care they thought they were entitled to. The former group needed urgent care after walking hundreds of kilometers, carrying with them infection and medical conditions. Most of these people Rafael had never met, and they had no access to a computer or an email account; so Rafael would be contacted by someone he knew in an NGO on their behalf. With the NGO's help, they would draft documents for Rafael so that he could file for an emergency injunction for medical care.

The latter group included people Rafael knew a little better. This included those who'd received notices from government officials asking for more paperwork or those who were simply denied the health care they needed. Rafael had started to get the hang of the system and recognized what he was up against. It was not only that nearly two-thirds of the people he met weren't eligible for care, it was also that those who *were* eligible had no way to figure out how to get care. His work was painstakingly slow. But every few days there would be a case that could not wait.

On that particular Monday, there was a case that couldn't wait. A five-year-old girl from Venezuela had come to Bogotá with her parents. Earlier that year, she'd had a kidney infection, which resulted in a surgery that removed her left kidney. Exposure to dirty water, long journeys, little food, and infection had taken a toll, and now her remaining kidney was failing. She was in pain and hanging on by a thread. The hospital wasn't providing her any emergency care. She wasn't a citizen, had no formal paperwork, wasn't in the national health care system (EPS),[2] and was told that she wasn't eligible for hospital care. One hospital receptionist told them that her case didn't count as an emergency. Another one said that there was no space in their hospital.

This girl reminded Rafael of his daughter, and though he hadn't met her personally, he felt her pain deep in his own bones. Rafael felt angry and helpless. He would constantly ask himself and everyone around him, "Where was all the foreign money for helping refugees going?" No answers. To him it felt as if the Venezuelan refugees were at the whim of NGOs, which were now an extension of the waste and corruption of the Venezuelan government.

Rafael went back to his email, carefully read the documents, and tried to figure out a way. He finally found one clause in the Colombian law that might help the girl. It was about filing for guardianship for medical care in case of a life-threatening emergency. The courts were supposed to respond to these filings within a few hours. In the past, Rafael's experience had been mixed, but he tried his luck. He drafted the document and followed up with a flurry of calls. He was soon given the standard response: "We will evaluate."

In the afternoon, he received a text. The girl would get the treatment she needed.

Henry tries to find medicine and staff for a local clinic

Soon after he'd returned to Juba from Malakan, Henry went to work at the hospital. As he passed through the main gate, he could see in the background the graveyard of equipment. This is where the hospital tossed old equipment, things that Henry had used some time ago but were now pieces of junk, as well as equipment sent by missionaries and their foundations in the United States and Europe that was broken even before it reached the hospital (equipment that everyone who pitched in felt good about). The equipment graveyard was a permanent part of the hospital landscape. And, like any other graveyard, it was growing. It was now visible from a distance.

Henry entered the hospital and turned down the corridors that led to his lab. He felt a clear drop in temperature inside, away from the scorching sun. He reached his lab and unlocked the door. He was the only one with a key to his lab. He was meticulous about his work space. Everything was organized, and the bottles were labeled. But now the workspace was bare. No real work had been done in the lab in months. There was nothing in the bottles that should have held consumables and supplies. The lab only had rubbing alcohol, and it was slowly evaporating.

Henry's community and members of his church in Malakan knew that he worked in a hospital lab. They'd asked him about COVID-19 and tests, but Henry had no answers to give. Some members of his church had dismissed the pandemic as a satanic curse, nothing that could affect the pious. Henry hadn't discouraged this view. He knew better but had nothing to offer as an alternative. When his congregants asked about the new virus, he deflected the conversation and asked them to pray, wash their hands, and stay positive.

The government in Juba, unlike Sudan in the north and Uganda in the south, was completely quiet on the issue of COVID-19. The ministry of health hadn't issued any statements either. From senior colleagues at the hospital, Henry heard that the WHO had sent South Sudan COVID-19 test kits. Had they made their way to Juba? Henry hadn't seen any. As a lab technician of the main hospital, he would be among the first to know about the test kits. He assumed he'd be trained to administer the test and/or analyze test results. Honestly, he was hoping that there'd be surplus supplies that he could save for other tests. But it had been completely quiet. His lab remained bare, except for rubbing alcohol.

As Henry sat at his desk, emotionally tired, he saw Dr. Julius walk by. Henry jumped up and rushed to catch the senior doctor in the hallway.

Dr. Julius and Henry had known each other for a decade. Dr. Julius was from the same tribe as Henry, and had some family in and around Wonduruba, and it was Dr. Julius who had gotten Henry his current job. He was a rich man, by Henry's standards, because he also had a private practice. Henry knew there was only few minutes to catch Dr. Julius before he left in the white Nissan Pathfinder to his private clinic.

"Good afternoon, Dr. Julius."

"Good afternoon, Henry. How was the trip?"

Henry told Dr. Julius about Solomon and about his visit to his village and the primary health care center there. Then he asked if there were some medicines available—perhaps in the store or extra medicines under Dr. Julius's care—that he could take back to Malakan to get the primary health care center functional again.

Dr. Julius thought for a second, looked at his watch, and told Henry to come the next day.

"I'll open the cabinet and see if there's anything we can spare," he told Henry.

This was promising and an answer different from the typical "let me see."

Henry thanked Dr. Julius and walked away, down the corridor that allowed Dr. Julius to get to his car without any patients in the waiting room seeing him. But then Henry turned back and ran toward Dr. Julius again. He had another question for him and knew it wasn't polite to shout his question, certainly not to Dr. Julius, a man who had trained in South Africa, spent time in the United Kingdom, and took his manners seriously. When Henry reached Dr. Julius, he asked his question in a hushed voice.

"Any news on the test kits?"

Dr. Julius looked at Henry curiously. "Yes, of course. We have some in the private hospital."

This was the same private hospital that almost exclusively served the expats working in international NGOs. The same NGOs that displayed billboards all over the country about their benevolence. The same NGOs that had promised to send the kits to the people of South Sudan.

Saida seeks care for her brother

Saida knew in her heart that Tanvir's case wasn't hopeless. She didn't have any scientific basis for her feeling, or experience working with people with mental health issues. She just had a feeling, which she trusted. She'd heard from neighbors that there were doctors outside the colony, working in more affluent areas, who could treat him and save him from attempting to take his life. But the problem wasn't treatment, it was access. Access required one of two things: having a formal national ID card or having money.[3] Saida and her family had neither.

Finding money for a private clinic was a nonstarter, so Saida chose to go the other route of obtaining a national ID. Tanvir was born in Pakistan after 1971, when the country split in two, and was therefore legally eligible for a national ID card. Pakistan had a birthright citizenship clause in its constitution; however, the legal cases of Bengalis born in Pakistan were still languishing in the courts.[4] They simply wanted what the state had agreed to give them. It wasn't hard to figure out why they weren't being treated fairly: the unscripted rules for Bengalis weren't based on the constitution but on the attitude of people all around Machar Colony.

Saida knew it would be a long process to obtain treatment, but she was eager to help her only brother. It gave her a sense of purpose in an otherwise depressing existence. Then, by a strange coincidence, soon after Saida had saved Tanvir from his second suicide attempt, she heard about a legal clinic in the colony that provided advice to people like her struggling with obtaining a national ID card. Saida couldn't remember how she'd heard about the new program. Was it a neighbor who'd told her? Did the volunteers come to her home? Did she see a poster somewhere? Or was it something else? In the chaos of her life, the sharp lines of memory and who, when, and what were always blurry. All she remembered was that she'd heard about an organization that could help.

Saida was initially skeptical. Why would anyone want to help? She was not well-traveled, but she knew her place in society. She was part of Machar Colony; to many people in Pakistan, she and her family were the mosquitos.

She asked her neighbor if they'd heard about the organization.

"There must be a catch. No one does anything for us without a motive," the neighbor said. Saida concurred.

Saida wasn't convinced that, in a place where no one cared who lived or died, anyone would care about their legal rights. Maybe it was another scam perpetrated by local con artists. There was always a new scam to fleece the poor. Saida had seen her share of such schemes.

She was also concerned that her brother's condition and his appearance would deter any lawyer willing to help. There were plenty of other, mentally and emotionally healthy, people who needed help. In a society where mental health ailments were taboo,[5] her brother's condition meant that his case was low on the list of priorities.

Saida debated whether or not to go to the legal clinic, her resolve to help her brother eventually won. Saida convinced herself there wasn't much to lose. They were already ostracized, and everyone knew that they had nothing left to offer or mortgage. Taking her brother to the legal clinic couldn't be more painful than seeing him slowly drift away from life.

She didn't tell her mother or ask anyone for advice. She'd made up her mind to go and talk to the staff at the legal clinic, and to take her brother with her.

The challenges of a separate health care system for refugees versus one national system

From the very beginning, refugee camps maintained a separate health care system (if one could call it a system at all) independent of the public health system.[6] Health services for refugees, in most low- and middle-income countries, are part of a distinct system that is often run by international NGOs using money from outside the country.[7] This system is often separate from the public hospitals that serve the citizens of the host country and is significantly different (in scope, staffing, and quality of care) from private hospitals,[8] which is where most members of international humanitarian agencies get treated.[9]

The model of health care services, operating exclusively for those in the camps, goes back as far as the camps themselves. Historically, health care was provided by nongovernmental and international humanitarian organizations, who worked directly or were contracted for their services by local governments, colonial powers, or international relief agencies.[10] These international organizations, whether the Near East Relief or the Red Cross, would bring European or American doctors, nurses, and professionals to run health care.[11] This model was created and supported by wealthier nations, and worked well with the overall goal of running the camp from afar.[12] The supply of humanitarian workers, who were often interested in doing what they considered their moral duty and God's work, was steady and supported through recruitment along various channels, including through a network of churches and missionary organizations in the United States and Europe.[13]

71

The supply of outside medical professionals also met a growing need. Camps that were increasing, both in number and in size, were facing repeated outbreaks of disease that had found willing hosts in weakened bodies due to conflict, injury, and malnutrition, combined with poor sanitation in and around the camps.[14] High population density made health conditions worse, while increasing the risk of rapid spread of infection.[15] Typhoid and cholera were becoming a routine occurrence,[16] though malaria, dysentery, and tuberculosis were not uncommon either.[17] Having outsiders be in charge of a matter as private as health, however, was not always a smooth process. Language and cultural barriers, conflict arising from social norms, and a contrasting worldview between the camp dwellers and the health care workers were among the issues that affected the camps.[18]

On the flip side, there were other issues related to the outsiders at times providing a more accurate assessment of the problems and corruption than what the local governments preferred to disclose. In the Pakistan camps in the immediate aftermath of the partition of India in 1947, details of the camp conditions were suppressed by the Pakistani government through an aggressive censorship policy. Personal accounts of missionary doctors and nurses—their letters and diaries—as well as medical reports provided a much richer analysis of the breakdown of the health system than what was available from the public health authorities in Pakistan.[19]

The colonial model or the "managed from a distance" approach, however, was not present in all camps. The camps that were of little interest to European and American powers were low on the politico-humanitarian list of priorities, and the displaced there were left to their own devices. For the camps that did not have colonial blessings, a more dynamic, hybrid model had organically grown. In this model, international organizations (e.g., the Red Cross), without the support of colonial powers or the United Nations, worked side-by-side with local volunteers and medical professionals. The camps in Pakistan were an example of a more integrated approach,[20] where there were more local doctors and plenty of trained and untrained volunteers.[21] It was, however, far from a perfect union. Similarly, in other camps there was an effort made to train local nurses, such as the training programs in Palestine in the 1930s.[22] Trust issues, however, have remained a staple and continue to this day. For example, in recent years there has been a strong push from international agencies for contraception and family planning (distinct from maternal health). These have been viewed with suspicion by local populations that may have doubts about the intentions of international organizations; consequently these policies have been met with resistance by the local refugee populations.[23]

Parallel Health Care System

The original model of a separate, exclusive health care system is still operational to a great extent with strong support in influential circles of international humanitarian financing.[24] The supporters for the idea of a refugee-specific health care system cite several reasons for its effectiveness. They argue that it provides possible and economically attractive job opportunities for refugees, creating employment in countries that otherwise would not employ refugees.[25] The jobs are not only for doctors and nurses but are within the entire medical and health ecosystem. An example often cited is UNRWA, an institution that supports clinics staffed largely by Palestinian refugees. UNRWA continues to provide both jobs and health care to the refugees who are otherwise denied both in the countries where they have been living for decades.[26] This is particularly true in Lebanon, where repeated economic downturns and legacies of the long civil war have made jobs for Palestinian refugees scarce.[27] In recent years, government policies have continued to decrease the number of possible jobs that Palestinians are able to apply for.[28]

Beyond employment, there are other strong, albeit less-discussed, reasons for preferring this model. A separate system allows for control over the lives of people who are denied integration and who the state feels need to be under its watchful eyes.[29] Everyone needs health care at some point in their lives, and refugees, who are otherwise unable to go to the public system or do not have the financial means to go to private hospitals, will rely on the system that caters only to refugees. Thus, even if the refugees are no longer living in camps, their movement and actions can still be tracked. From a logistics point of view, the separate system model also enables a clear channel for movement of money and resources, from rich countries and the international agencies, to concrete places, as opposed to systems that are complex, organic, and harder to navigate for outsiders.[30] It makes accounting a lot easier.

In recent years, with an increased emphasis on metrics and data[31] (as a means to measure "impact"), the separate system allows for analysis and the customary pat on the back—something that would be messy and difficult for integrated systems. As David Keen points out, metrics allow for accountability of NGOs that are more designed toward donors (upwards) then the communities they serve (downwards). Emphasis on metrics and data has created a warped sense of accomplishment and impact that is self-serving as opposed to one that aims to understand and analyze the real change on the ground.[32] This incentivizes NGOs to provide a favorable review of their own activities, whereas the reality may be different. A recent study pointed out that in a self-evaluation of thirty-five Dutch NGOs focused on relief, not one came up with a predominantly negative evaluation.[33] While *impact* has become a buzzword lately, it has led to little changes in the way things are actually practiced.

The separate health care system, put in place for refugees, has been guided by two factors from its inception: control and impermanence. Governments, on whose lands the refugees are housed, have always had strong interest in maintaining absolute control of the camps and of the lives of those who live in them.[34] These governments have been concerned not only about integration (and its political cost) but also about burdening local hospitals, as well as the spread of infection from outsiders who were viewed through a lens of suspicion and racism.[35] A separate health care system can appease local governments (or colonial powers in charge of local affairs) that control the land and access to the camps.

The second factor guiding the separate health care system has been the (incorrect) assessment that camps are meant to be temporary,[36] and hence the health care system needed to cater to this reality. The nature of camps, building materials, and insistence on projecting an image of impermanence (chapter 2) is very much part of that worldview. As a result, the systems are often designed with a similar framework, as humanitarian emergencies, with an approach that had a stronger influence of conflict medicine or public health emergencies than attending to the health care needs of a protracted crisis. Public health research focused on the refugee crisis continues to view refugee camps through the lens of a humanitarian disaster.[37]

The presence and outsized role of international agencies, whose expertise was largely in managing emergencies, further drove the system toward a particular kind of health care that was more focused on epidemics, outbreaks, physical trauma, injury, and related emergencies.[38] This model relies on the rotation mechanism of expat experts coming to the camp through international agencies, thereby further adding to the underlying assumption that camps are temporary humanitarian agencies. The health challenges for those in the camps, however, are not reflective of a temporary humanitarian emergency.[39]

The camps, in many parts of the world, have stayed in a permanent state of impermanence for decades.[40] This means that there are not only multiple generations of people living in the camps,[41] but there are also new groups of people added, as babies are born, children become adolescents, girls become mothers, and young people age and need care as elderly members of the community.[42] The health system, however, has remained rigid and incapable of flexibility and growth. While there has often been an emphasis on maternal and child health, care for the elderly or palliative care is often completely absent from the camps.[43]

Schooling

The presence of the camps for extended periods also creates the need (and demand) for schooling and specialty health care.[44] This demand

and need is distinct from the needs after a natural disaster emergency, which doesn't create a need for new schools or large, multispecialty health centers. Thus while camp-based systems are often designed for impermanence, the demand reflects a different reality.[45] Meeting this demand means creating new structures (physical and institutional) and new (and continuously inflating) bureaucracy to manage these growing needs. While both health and education are considered basic services, are connected on several levels (e.g., nutrition, awareness, vaccinations, etc.[46]), and have been among the priorities of international agencies, the response from local authorities, often in partnership with international agencies, has been markedly different.

Despite being grouped together as priorities, education and health care have been approached very differently in the camps. In some camps, the issue of schooling, initially ignored due to the insistence on impermanence and treating the situation as a short-term humanitarian crisis, eventually got political attention based on concerns about potential extremism, indoctrination of vulnerable communities, and terrorism. The Afghan camps in Pakistan represent this evolution of policy.[47]

The typical rotation of outside doctors and nurses, who come for a few weeks or months and then leave, couldn't work in schools. But there is often strong resistance to providing integrated education to refugee children in local schools.[48] The sources of this resistance are several. The government doesn't value integration as a meaningful policy, and the local population (who are often driven by a sense of racial or economic superiority or a sense of anxiety about loss of essential services) sees refugees as outsiders and don't want their children's schools, which are already poorly resourced, to stretch the human and infrastructural resources further.

The vacuum for schooling is occasionally filled by local nongovernmental institutions including local religious schools (e.g., madrassas that support male students in Pakistan including Afghan refugees[49]).

At other times schooling for refugee children is provided during evening shifts in existing local schools.[50] Neither of these models has worked well. In the case of madrassas, there are few options for girls, and local authorities have little control over the curriculum. In the case of evening classes, refugee children are taught by teachers who are tired, underpaid, and disincentivized to work. Because the schools are not within walking distance from the camps, the refugee children need to take school buses; but the transportation system is unreliable and fraught with financial and logistical challenges.[51]

Complex Relationship with the Local Community

While the broader issue of control has continued to influence the evolution of health care, the reality is that creating and sustaining a health care system has been influenced not only by available resources (human and financial, within and outside the country) but also by the real and perceived responses of the local community.[52] The relationship between the local community and those who are forced to live in camps is complex.[53] This spectrum of this complexity goes from business transactions and family relationships, on one end, to insecurity, xenophobia, and violence, on the other.[54] While this sense is exaggerated when the refugees, stateless communities, or internally displaced persons belong to a different ethnicity, race, or religion, even communities that share the same heritage and culture (for example, Syrians in Lebanon or Pashtun Afghans in Pakistan's Pashtun tribal regions) are not immune to a hostile response.[55] An example is the tension between Palestinians who moved to Gaza (from areas that became part of Israel) and those Palestinians who already lived there.[56] The same tension plays out frequently in the case of the internally displaced persons.

The behavior of local communities in those regions represents shades of trust and mistrust, not only toward the outsider but also toward their own government.[57] This has led to the creation, and experimentation, with various models and systems of health care.

ǀ Two Separate Systems versus One Integrated System

The reaction of the local host community to a separate health care system for refugees has been mixed and at times contradictory. On one hand, adding refugee patients to existing, overburdened hospitals has created an outcry and an increase in xenophobia, anxiety, and calls for expulsion of the outsiders.[58] These objections have appeared in newspaper articles, opinion pieces, television programs, and more recently on social media.[59] Capitalizing on the notion that refugees may bring novel diseases or negatively affect the local population has energized anti-immigration groups in multiple countries.[60]

An integrated health care system has provided the anti-immigration and anti-refugee groups with an argument that refugees are making it harder for the local communities to seek health care in their own hospitals and are taking away the rights of the locals and taxpayers (a term referred by some as *medical xenophobia*[61]). Without any substantial historical evidence, these groups have tried to argue that before the arrival of the refugees, the hospitals were able to provide quality care. That environment of access and quality, according to this argument, changed with the arrival of refugees, who tend to be sicker and poorer and hence in greater and more frequent need of care.[62] These groups, and individuals who support this argument, would point to overburdened and unclean hospitals that show a collapsed health system that works for no one, not for the refugees and not for the locals. These groups further argue that refugees should not be allowed to use, at public expense, public health care centers. This argument, in many ways, mirrors the economic argument used by anti-immigration groups suggesting that outsiders take away jobs from locals[63] and hence shouldn't be allowed in.

On the other hand, the model of two separate systems has its own detractors, curiously sometimes within the same (or similar) anti-immigration or anti-refugee communities. Their argument is based on the perceived notion that while the locals and host communities rely on exhausted, stretched, fragmented, and poorly run health care systems, refugees may get access to additional services not available to the local population.[64] They are aware that refugee clinics are often run by international aid agencies that employ doctors (albeit temporarily) who may be better trained than local doctors. There is some merit to this argument since the local health care system is often in complete disarray and, from a distance, the health care provided to refugees seems more structured and organized. In Jordan, for example, the local residents of an Azraq village wanted to register as refugees since the care provided to Syrians was far superior to the care available to local residents surrounding the new camp.[65]

This argument is further extended to suggest that locals are being discriminated against, while refugees are benefitting from the support of international agencies.

Quality of medicines is also cited as an argument against separate systems, especially in countries that have a long history of poor quality, substandard, and outright fake medicines. While poor quality medicines exist for many reasons—including inadequate local regulation, issues in manufacturing and storage, lack of oversight, and corruption, as well as diplomatic and commercial pressure from countries with a large manufacturing base—the presence and prevalence of medicines that are counterfeit and substandard makes the local community distrustful of those patients who don't have to buy or consume medicines made locally. Those who are wary of separate systems argue that while the host communities have access to only locally made medicines, which are neither free nor of good quality, the refugees get medicines that are imported from abroad, which are of superior quality and are offered free of cost. Thus, they would argue, refugees, who do not belong in the country in the first place and bring in all kinds of evil, from terrorism to disease, get preferential treatment compared to local residents who are bona fide citizens.

Interestingly, this argument, which created hostility against refugees enjoying better medicine quality and by extension better and preferential care, has found support not only in the anti-immigrant and anti-refugee communities but also among local pharmaceutical companies and businesses associated with these companies.[66] Realizing that their businesses were being undermined by better quality imports and that the international agencies weren't *allowed* to buy from them, local pharmaceutical companies in several refugee hosting countries started lobbying the local governments. This argument received so much support that several governments, including Uganda, Jordan, and Lebanon, required international agencies working in their countries to procure their medicines *only* from local suppliers and not import them directly. The UNHCR and affiliated agencies eventually had to comply with the new rules, regardless of how they felt about having to procure medicines likely of inferior quality.

While the tension between the local residents and the internally displaced is less pronounced than tensions between local communities and refugees who are non-citizens, the presence of a system that is exclusive to a particular group (refugees or IDPs), funded and supported by international agencies, is likely to cause mistrust and frustration among the local residents if the quality of their own system is inferior to the camp's system.[67]

The result of this tussle between whether to have two separate systems or one integrated system is that there ends up being *no real system* in place for refugees; health care access is often through a patchwork of short-term policies that are often contradictory and constantly evolving.[68] This patchwork system is also not resilient to social pressures, and services can be disrupted because of local hostility toward the displaced communities. For example, in case of a conflict, the entire international staff may leave, resulting in a collapse of services for the vulnerable community. In instances when donor funding falls short of demand, which has happened often in Yemen, IDPs are left without essential life-saving care.[69] Another dimension of the patchwork system is that it is often redundant in some services and lacking in others.[70] This redundancy is often due to the interests of international donor agencies that may prioritize specific goals and provide substantial financial resources for them (e.g., family planning) while ignoring other services (e.g., postpartum depression[71]) that may be related to the same overarching goal (i.e., maternal and child health). With a top-down approach, where development programs are prioritized by outside funding agencies, there is often a gap between what the community may actually need and what services are offered.[72] Because international funding agencies have specific priorities, the system creates silos and vertical programs that are not connected to other programs or service, as opposed to more holistic programs[73]. For example, funding to improve the quality of medicines may come from an agency focused on malaria control, and would prioritize testing of malaria medicines, while ignoring the quality of other medicines.

Primary Health Care Centers

The main purpose of a primary health care unit is to be the first point of care. It is meant for checkup, consultation, and dispensing of medicines for common ailments; it is designed to be a guide for subsequent specialized care for those who need it. Theoretically, the primary care centers are supposed to be connected to other parts of the system, working through referrals, which would allow patients to get adequate and appropriate care. The primary care center only works well as part of a larger system rather than operating in a vacuum.[74] In theory, patients in the camps or urban informal settlements who can't be provided adequate care through the primary care center would be sent to secondary and tertiary care centers that provide care through an established protocol and agreement, relying on ID and insurance cards. Primary care centers have some basic facilities, and often have an in-house pharmacy, but they are, by design, not capable of addressing emergencies, urgent care, specialized treatments, or surgery.

Primary health care is increasingly viewed as a cornerstone of a robust system of health care provision for refugees and displaced communities. This evolution in ideas and policies for forcibly displaced communities reflects broader thematic changes in public health practice seen in the last century. The initial camps lacked a centralized mechanism and had little coordination, and care provisions remained ad hoc. In Pakistan's refugee camps in 1947–1948, there was no centralized mechanism to provide care or to gather or disseminate information.[75] Various groups did what they thought was right, without working with other groups. For example, in Pakistan there was an effort to control epidemics but no real efforts in prevention or sanitation.[76] Similarly, in other camps, there were fumigation and quarantine facilities and even some education initiatives, but they were not linked to any system-level efforts to improve health outcomes among refugees.[77] Health care was also defined narrowly. For example, issues of violence against women, an issue that had reached epidemic proportions in Pakistan with as many as 50,000 women being abducted and subjected to unspeakable violence, was dealt with as a security and law-and-order issue,[78] but no care was available to deal with the trauma of the survivors.

The approach changed as the field of public health evolved in the twentieth century with the emergence of primary care as a central pillar of the system.[79] This changing face of public health theory, scholarship, and practice, and the increased emphasis on primary health, has also affected how care provision is imagined for refugees. Starting in the mid-1960s, camps began to rely more on primary health care centers (or basic health services, as they were sometimes referred[80]). The theoretical role of primary care is evident from how camps are built, constructed, and imagined today. Even in urban slums where stateless communities live, the fractured health system starts with a primary care clinic[81] that is often supported by a foreign donor.[82]

Today, most camps have one, or in some cases several, primary health care units that are near the camp, though there are several gaps in information and guidance on how to operate and organize these primary care facilities.[83]

Staffing of primary health centers continues to be a challenge due to a limited supply of staff willing (or able) to work in these camps.[84] This is not only an issue for foreign staff but also for staff from local host communities. For international staff, there is often a short supply of people willing to work in difficult conditions for a long period of time. Their salary costs can also be a significant challenge. Furthermore, foreign staff are dependent on the local host country for entry visas and staying privileges. In addition, there are concerns that language and cultural barriers[85] may exacerbate friction among the residents of the camps and the health officials. Likewise, issues of racism or elitism cannot be downplayed.[86] Working in camps is not seen as a prudent move for those interested in career advancement.[87]

There are other underappreciated challenges as well when it comes to staffing primary health centers. For example, while the centers may be located near camps so that patients can walk to them, many staff members don't live near the health centers. This means that centers may not be open to handle health issues that happen after normal work hours, on weekends, or holidays.[88] In addition health centers aren't equipped to provide emergency care, which means a family has to take the patient directly to a hospital, which could be far away and expensive (and require upfront payment).

Housing for staff—especially international staff who are paid attractive salaries—can also be a complicated issue. Creating housing that is far superior to the conditions in the camps, or in more secure and elite neighborhoods, drives home a sense of inequality between staff and patients. In the absence of good housing, the likelihood of attracting qualified medical staff becomes a challenge. In certain cases, such as in Yemen IDP camps, medical aid is provided via mobile clinics[89] rather than in fixed structures near the camps. This means that near the IDP camps, no continuous medical service is available,[90] and doctors and medical professionals remain inaccessible on short notice. While the mobile clinics are staffed and equipped with medicines and diagnostics, their availability varies and may be completely suspended due to political and financial constraints, making it impossible for residents of the camp to get any medical help during a time of urgent need.[91] In the case of Pakistan and its stateless Bengali population, none of the staff working in Machar Colony lives near the colony. Given the conditions of the colony, living in or near the colony would be unimaginable.[92]

Unfortunately, there is a wide gap in perception regarding primary care units. Care providers—doctors, nurses, and midwives—have a different view than the refugees and the forcibly displaced about what the health center is and what it can do. In the absence of a connected system, patients often view the primary care center as a comprehensive care center. In the Adjumani camps, in northern Uganda near the South Sudan border, the primary care center routinely gets patients who need specialized care and are therefore turned away. In Machar Colony, pregnancy-related complications are often brought to the maternity clinic, which has no capacity for complicated surgery. When expectations are not met, patients often go to underground clinics and unlicensed professionals who promise a more comprehensive solution to their health needs.

Mismatch of expectations and perceptions is not the only challenge. The primary care units, in camps and in informal settlements, also continue to underperform in several ways, such as long wait times, high patient volume, misdiagnosis, poor patient experience, lack of essential medicines, and lack of functioning diagnostic equipment.[93] This near-permanent underperformance is related to infrastructural, human, financial, and medical resources and the center's ability to replenish these resources at regular intervals and on short notice. In some cases funds are allocated for initial construction but not for upkeep and maintenance. Hence it is common to see abandoned health center buildings due to lack of funds. A center's ability to provide care varies with its ability to replenish its resources. There is also a clear decline in performance with time. It's not unusual that, within a few months of its opening, a new center looks like a shell of itself—a building remains standing but has no real ability to provide care. With the passage of time and limited resources, primary health centers often become structures with broken equipment and no medicines.

The issue of equipment maintenance is an important one for global health, in general, but is largely an underappreciated barrier to performance.[94] Primary care centers often don't have sophisticated equipment to begin with, and even simple equipment (weighing scales, refrigerators, etc.) routinely break down and require extensive paperwork and bureaucracy for them to be repaired.

An additional challenge facing a parallel system is that primary care centers have their own separate governance mechanisms[95] and are disconnected from the main health system; therefore they are unable to tap into the human resources of the main system. For example, when equipment needs repair, technicians working in the public system of the host country cannot simply come and fix it. Technical personnel are already limited in low- and middle-income countries, and then layers of bureaucracy makes fixing equipment even more challenging. Since health care centers near camps in a parallel system do not report directly to the central public health system, they often have their own processes for maintenance (that is, if they have any process at all). These health centers therefore have to look to the private sector, which can be expensive. With limited funds, there are long delays in fixing essential equipment. The prevalence of broken equipment is often a major source of frustration for both staff and patients, but this issue fails to capture the attention of international agencies. Recently, there has been some promotion of vocational training in maintaining medical devices, but that effort has been ad hoc[96] and hasn't received the necessary investment. Equipment maintenance has also suffered from a lack of interest from international agencies, which are often concerned with metrics associated with patient data rather than with strengthening the system. Furthermore, in low- and middle-income countries, there are few vocational training institutes with a focus on medical technologies.[97]

Primary health units and their staff often deal with health problems they can't address. For example, health emergencies, such as complications during pregnancies, are not uncommon.[98] Yet, they often occur due to poor access to antenatal care, undiagnosed underlying conditions, poor diet, exposure to infection, and high levels of anxiety.[99] In addition severe poverty and a male-dominated, male-centered culture with expectations of married women to bear many (male) children disincentivizes women from seeking care early on.[100] Women are also dependent on their male relatives to take them to the clinics. Resulting complications—that could have been addressed early on through consultation and awareness[101]—often can't be handled by a primary care clinic.

Primary health centers are neither created, nor run, as places with proper infection control mechanisms, and they often lack basic services including water, electricity, and ventilation,[102] further undermining their ability to provide quality care.[103] In refugee clinics, it is not unusual for patients to wait hours in cramped environments with other patients who may be sick or infectious. As a result, communities develop a sense of frustration and distrust toward the formal system and seek health care elsewhere, including in informal and unlicensed care settings.[104] There is often a high dependence on pharmacies (legitimately licensed or otherwise), which fill the vacuum created by a poorly functioning primary health care system. Pharmacy staff usually aren't trained in pharmaceutical sciences but develop a general sense through experience or internships, and they provide information, medical advice, and medicines without the need for a prescription. This is particularly true for antibiotics, which serve multiple purposes, from fever reduction to infection cure. Most of all, antibiotics, even when not effective or useful, provide the patient with psychological comfort for getting some kind of treatment.[105]

Beyond pregnancy and post-delivery care, the demand for chronic disease management continues to be poorly addressed by primary health care units. Mental health, for example, has gotten far more attention in academic circles, prestigious publications, and elite conferences than in actual clinics.[106] In camp communities, mental health problems are often addressed by faith healers, unlicensed professionals, and willing pharmacists who prescribe medicines as they see fit. Diabetes, similarly, is a major problem, but lack of early diagnosis, subsidized regular testing, and affordable medicines makes it a debilitating challenge for refugees.[107] Recent data on cancer also shows that early detection doesn't happen, so cancers that are treatable often metastasize and become a near-certain death sentence.[108] Unfortunately, even respectful and effective palliative care for those with terminal diseases is practically nonexistent.[109]

Data Management

A well-run primary care center needs to be able to share medical data and transfer it securely to the next point in the health system, thereby avoiding redundancies and the costs associated with them, and ensuring that the provider in the secondary or tertiary system is aware of the medical history of the patient. In a weak system, little data collection and sharing happens to connect the primary care center to other units in the system; therefore tests may be repeated and additional expenses incurred. Unfortunately, in the health centers in and around camps, the issue of data capture and recordkeeping is both archaic and insecure.[110] On one end, data capture mechanisms continue to rely on ledgers, registers, and handwritten entries, and on the other end, the burden is often on the patient to provide all data about prior visits. Data quality remains generally poor.[111] In some cases immunization cards are issued to mothers, but that information is not copied or stored anywhere else; or if it is stored, it's hard to track down on short notice.[112] Loss of an immunization card, which is not uncommon among camp residents, results in confusion and frustration for both the patient and the provider. With rotating doctors, lack of information means the patient has to rely on their own memory, regurgitate information, or simply guess about prior visits.

The solution to data management is not as simple as creating an electronic health records system. Beyond the significant financial investment needed to create such a system, there are legitimate trust issues among vulnerable communities about their personal information.[113] Communities already wary of surveillance continue to be concerned about who will have access to their data and whether data capture for health means that the host government (which is already unhappy about their presence) may decide to use this data to deport or arrest them. While there is often giddy excitement in international aid agencies about the newest data analytics method, little has been done to create a sense of trust among the refugees and the forcibly displaced.[114]

Security Concerns

The health system is not merely impacted by lack of funds, poor maintenance, and staff turnover. Additional challenges come from physical attacks on health care staff and centers.[115] In areas where there is continued conflict, health care centers, run by international NGOs or by the local host population, are routinely targeted by a variety of armed groups.[116] Health centers may be the target or may be caught in the crossfire. In Yemen, for example, MSF (Médecins Sans Frontières; Doctors without Borders) centers have suffered[117] due to bombing by the Saudi-led coalition, and other health care professionals have suffered from the Houthi combatants. Similar incidents have been seen in the Democratic Republic of the Congo (DRC), Syria, South Sudan, and Afghanistan, to name a few.[118] Data from the last five years suggest that on average there have been over a hundred attacks per year on health care centers and staff.[119] Limited security is provided to health care centers near camps and settlements.

Security concerns deter health workers, nurses, midwives, and doctors from working in these settings, further disrupting care. Security concerns also affect large international agencies working in the area. With attacks on hospital facilities in Afghanistan and Yemen and elsewhere, the impact on providing care has been severe.[120] These security issues not only disrupt care in continued programs (e.g., vaccinations) but also affect the physical architecture and infrastructure of the facility, making them inoperable for long periods and draining already meager resources.[121] Providing security is also a real cost that has to be calculated when thinking of installing a new facility, further diminishing money for actual health care services.[122]

Health Care for IDPs and Stateless Persons

While the parallel system's original design was for refugees, the model has attached itself to the broader idea of displaced persons.[123] Thus one can find poorly staffed and nearly bare primary health centers even among the camps for internally displaced persons in various parts of the world from Yemen and Pakistan to the DRC.[124] The internally displaced communities often get caught up in a model that wasn't designed with them in mind, and one that is primarily operational due to funds from outside agencies such as IOM or UNICEF. In some instances, the primary health centers for IDPs might even be in worse condition than the ones in refugee camps for a variety of reasons, including lack of support from international agencies and limited international media attention.

The worst system for health care access, however, is for those who are stateless.[125] Even international agencies are unlikely to invest, citing their lack of a mandate, along with resistance from the local government (for a variety of reasons ranging from racism to suspicion of the stateless). Despite the contextual experiences that are important to recognize and vary from one geography to another, the overall experience of internally displaced communities and the stateless has several similarities to the experience of refugees.[126] In terms of the primary care available, all three groups do worse than the resident population. Racism, exclusion, and distrust work in synergy with a dysfunctional or nonexistent primary care system. Ultimately, it often matters little whether the people in need of care cross an international border, are displaced from their home and move to another part of the country, or are simply struck off the list of who gets to be a citizen.

The absence of a trustworthy and reliable system means that communities often try to manage their ailments themselves through guesswork, self-medication,[127] word-of-mouth advice, and traditional healers.[128] Most displaced people (particularly the stateless and the migrants who cross the border without formal documentation) don't have access to subsidized care, but even those who do may find the hospitals overburdened and that they are asked to pay out of their own pocket for basic services (that range from diagnostic tests to medicines).[129] They may be forced to seek care in a private hospital, where the high costs may send them further into debt,[130] and which may eventually involve extortion and harassment.

Driven by anxiety of living in the camps, or the lack of opportunity to provide for their families, or seeing the camp as another tool of control over their lives, many displaced people choose to live in urban areas among the local population rather than in a camp. While there is a disincentive to leave the camps (e.g., not having a nearby primary care clinic, even a poorly functioning one), the number of people who leave has continued to increase significantly.[131] In some cases, like in Colombia, there are no formal camps to begin with. However, urban environments and high-density residences create their own challenges in both chronic and infectious diseases. The forcibly displaced have to depend on health care services provided by public hospitals, private institutions, or NGOs.[132]

It wouldn't be fair to argue that there is no effort from any state whatsoever. However, state efforts can fall short or may help only the first group of arrivals, while subsequent groups can't get the care they need.[133] The insurance system created for Venezuelan migrants arriving in Colombia was designed to provide them affordable, quality care. However, it suffered from two immediate challenges. First, the system became quickly overwhelmed.[134] The formal documentation needed to enroll migrants was often unavailable.[135] The insurance instruments created for these communities were unable to cope with the influx of migrants.[136] This chaos created long periods when those who needed care didn't have any insurance to get it, which led to confusion and frustration among all parties. Second, the system worked only for those who were formally registered. As the system became overburdened, registering new arrivals stopped.[137] Thus a number of those who came through the proper mechanisms and had formal documentations did not have care for a period of time.

The overburdening of hospitals by "outsiders" and increasing xenophobia has led to the growing chorus of voices within Colombia to "send the Venezuelans back."[138] There is also a power dynamic at play that manifests itself at care facilities. Despite possessing an official and formal right to care, a Venezuelan may be denied care due to xenophobia, and there is little formal recourse available to them to address it. In case of denial of care, migrants need the services of a willing lawyer. The matter to adjudicate often goes to courts, which themselves may be overwhelmed.

| COVID-19

The political climate and a rapid rise in nationalism and nativism in the last decade has created a declining interest globally in refugee acceptance and integration.[139] The rise of anti-immigration sentiment in rich countries has led to an emphasis on repatriation and stronger curbs on movement. These challenges were further exacerbated by the global novel coronavirus pandemic (COVID-19).

In the midst of the global pandemic, international and local support for refugees has declined further.[140] While this trend already existed, it became even more prominent in the COVID-19 era. Access to basic services has slowed to a trickle for the forcibly displaced. Both rapid tests and vaccinations (when they became available) reached displaced communities much later than local resident citizens.[141] While there were some exceptions (e.g., Jordan[142]), national policies on testing, reporting, and vaccinating excluded refugees and stateless persons.[143] In Pakistan, for example, the Bengali stateless communities were initially denied vaccines[144] and were only allowed to get vaccinations several months after they became available for Pakistani citizens. Even then, there were barriers for Bengali stateless persons to actually getting vaccinated. For example, in order to be eligible, Bengali stateless persons had to have a mobile phone in their name (which itself requires a national ID card). Similarly the vaccination centers were often far away and difficult to reach by public transportation within a reasonable time.[145] In other places like Yemen, the government denied the existence of COVID-19 altogether.[146] In other parts of Yemen and in Afghanistan, where there are a large number of IDPs, the already fragmented health system was decimated by the combination of a recent famine, other infectious diseases like cholera, and COVID-19.[147]

Repatriation

During the COVID-19 global pandemic, repatriation, which had always been on the agenda, became the top item.[148] Countries, like Pakistan, closed their borders with Afghanistan with greater enforcement and at the same time encouraged refugees to return.[149] Host countries that benefited from international aid to keep refugees and used part of those funds for their own development, have fewer international resources that can be tapped into for their own development and spending. For some, it has provided an opportunity to send the refugees back; for others it led to closing their doors. Uganda, for example, soon after the declaration of the global pandemic, closed its borders for new South Sudanese refugees.[150]

Those who are forced, coerced, or nudged into repatriation can find themselves accessing a health care system that is weaker and more fragmented than the one they left behind.[151] There is anxiety about the security and safety of the situation being no better than when these communities originally left. In addition to health care needs, people are seriously concerned about employment, food, and education as a result of the collapse of the physical and institutional infrastructure, destruction of lands that were used for cultivation, and an exodus of professionals.

Those who repatriate find themselves in situations that may have even fewer resources than the camps. There are—like in the camps—primary care centers, but they remain empty of both staff and supplies. The investment for rebuilding in countries like South Sudan is minimal and slow to arrive.[152] In many cases the governments—that were previously labeled corrupt or hostile—are still in power, and now the international community has learned to accept them and are no longer holding them to account. For example, in 2021 Syria was among the select few countries elected to the WHO executive board.[153]

The repatriated communities return home to find that the system that they desperately need to work for them needs to be rebuilt not just strengthened. These countries had weak health systems to begin with, as a result of colonialism, corruption, and/or lack of international and domestic accountability. With the advent of the crises that led to forced displacement, public health systems suffered badly. Doctors, nurses, and health professionals were either targeted and killed, or they left the country. Local manufacturing was weak to begin with, and with impacted supply chains, the ability of the system to replenish took a further hit. With little interest in rebuilding by the international community, there is a concern among the staff of humanitarian organizations about safety.[154] As a result, the number of internationally supported clinics are few. With few local experts around, there is a clear vacuum in health services. In this situation, many may choose to return to the camps.[155]

Current Situation

At the time of this writing (2023), Afghanistan is the starkest example of a weak system put under further stress by near complete dependence on international aid, security concerns for foreign workers, and a risk of widespread epidemics.[156] The rapid withdrawal of US and NATO forces and the subsequent reemergence of the Taliban brought with it a series of interconnected humanitarian challenges that is, by some estimates, even worse than the humanitarian crisis in Yemen that started with the Saudi-led military operations. In the aftermath of

US withdrawal, only a small fraction of the people who wanted to leave the country were able to. The general chaos of the last two weeks of August 2021 prioritized the evacuation of US military personnel, the diplomatic staff of US and Western embassies, and Afghans who were well-connected or more affluent.[157] While it's reasonable to assume that many others may have wanted to leave, most Afghans did not have a passport. With the Kabul airport barely functioning, flights were few and expensive, and the land borders with Iran and Pakistan were heavily guarded. So far, the two countries have allowed a very small number of people to pass through.[158] The government of Pakistan has also taken a position to not allow significant numbers of refugees, a position that has substantial domestic support.[159]

As a result of these events, there are millions of Afghans who are displaced from their homes within their own country. This crisis has serious health implications. Years of conflict, poverty, corruption, and mismanagement by successive governments, combined with the United States and other Western countries blocking aid (or even access to Afghan sovereign funds), has resulted in near-famine conditions.[160] The health care situation was precarious to begin with, but it's made worse by the continued departure of doctors, nurses, and other health professionals. For the few hospitals that do exist and are functioning, their operation is made more difficult by the limited supplies able to reach the country. There are also security concerns, and distrust of the Taliban government, on the minds of outside health care professionals. It was reported in December 2021 that Afghanistan is facing a series of epidemics[161] and not just COVID-19. Malaria, dengue, measles, and typhoid, and widespread malnutrition have destroyed homes and families, while the complete absence of reliable aid is making the chance of recovery almost impossible. While there have been some calls from public health professionals, diplomats, and politicians (most notably from Pakistan[162]), the aid reaching Afghans has been far from sufficient.[163] Furthermore, the recent policy by the Taliban authorities barring any women from working in NGOs is likely to have a devastating impact on health, safety, and well-being of millions of citizens.[164]

The situation in Afghanistan, while disturbing, is not unique. It is part of the long pattern of donor dependence, corruption, fixation on cosmetic features, and lack of attention to building a resilient health system. The price of collapse of the system is always paid by its weakest members.

Chapter 4
Trusted Social Networks
Help Navigate the System

Rafael discovers the
value of trusted social networks

After living in Colombia for a few years, Rafael discovered it was a country that couldn't make up its mind. The contradictions were everywhere. It wasn't only the landscape—which went from the warm beaches of the Caribbean coast to the dense Amazon jungle where trees and bushes twisted their stems so they could catch the elusive rays of light. It wasn't only the history—the city of Bogotá defied all rules of how cities were historically established, typically near a coast or natural stream, and were developed over time. Bogotá was surrounded by mountains, and the city's air quality was among the worst in the continent; yet, it remained vibrant and in a permanent state of growth for well over four centuries. For Rafael, Colombian state and politics, like Bogotá, did not follow any predictions, norms, or rules.

Colombia had gone through decades of civil war that had started before Rafael was even born. There had been several peace treaties with the usual confident and bold headlines, but it wasn't clear to Rafael, as an outsider, whether the nation was at peace with itself.[1] Former FARC (Revolutionary Armed Forces of Colombia) soldiers who'd somehow survived, their sympathizers, and millions of ordinary people displaced or scarred by the war were all citizens and enemies at the same time. The people in the big cities, who'd been repeatedly targeted by the FARC, wanted to live in peace and often talked about harmony and forgiveness. Yet, they wanted their neighbors to be like them, and not be people who may have lived in enemy territory or may have had sympathies for the FARC in a former life. The citizens of cities chanted slogans of coexistence, as long as coexistence meant the "others" lived somewhere far from their homes. It wasn't easy for Rafael to figure out what people actually wanted. Yet, there was something charming about these contradictions. The unpredictability was authentic and attractive. This city of contradictions had started to grow on him.

The state's contradictory policies were just as impossible to figure out when it came to refugees and migrants. Plans announced by the government in early 2021 to give long-term visas to Venezuelans in the country[2] were hailed around the world as progressive and inclusive. There were congratulatory tweets and Facebook posts. Some had even hailed this as the most progressive and humane policy, yet Rafael knew firsthand that the reality on the ground was different. He'd read some of the stories and was bombarded with questions from Venezuelans in Colombia about the new rules. He knew better than to simply fall for another scheme that was likely, in the end, to do little for those he met every day. He told his friends to hold off the celebrations for now.

The announcement about long-term visas for Venezuelans came at one of the peaks of the COVID-19 pandemic in Colombia. Like the rest of the world, the poor and the uninsured were doing worse than those who had financial means.[3] There was some discussion about the importance of getting care to the Venezuelans, not because it was the humane thing to do but because sick Venezuelans suffering from COVID-19 were a risk to Colombians.[4] But Rafael's network, from all across Colombia, was telling him that hospitals in big cities continued to refuse care to Venezuelans. It didn't matter what the announcement from the president's office had said. The big office cared little about small people.

In the previous few weeks, Rafael had gotten to know a young family whose son probably had cancer. "Probably" because the boy couldn't get diagnosed. His parents had repeatedly taken him to the nearest hospital but were told that, as Venezuelan migrants, they were eligible for *some* urgent care, but their case, based on hospital definitions, was not urgent enough. The Venezuelan family couldn't argue effectively about definitions of urgency and their legal rights, so they got in touch with Rafael for help. He'd filed for court injunction and had gotten some traction with the courts, but it was too slow. The courts didn't feel that the boy's condition was life-threatening, and hence they weren't bound to respond immediately. After some time, the family stopped contacting Rafael. This typically meant that things either got much better or much worse. In most cases, it was the latter. In this case, Rafael's worst fears turned out to be true.

Not long after this case, another young woman, who reached out to Rafael through her relatives, was told by the receptionist at a hospital in Bogotá that she couldn't be seen by anyone. No doctor, no nurse came to see her when she complained of stomach pain. She was filtered out at the first point of entry at the hospital. There was an impenetrable wall between her and the care she needed. Rafael was seeing such walls everywhere.

Having no formal immigration documents meant no insurance; no insurance meant no care at most hospitals. Determining if the need was urgent was subjective. At least 60 percent of Venezuelans in Colombia (and nearly all Venezuelans who reach out to Rafael) are without formal registration.[5] This means routine denials for care. The health care system in Colombia is arguably free, except for many Venezuelans who need it most.

Rafael's task was to find clarity in this chaos, to find a path in this maze. A maze that changed its shape in time and space. COVID-19 had created new challenges (with high numbers of infections) and new opportunities (a discussion about getting the undocumented some care, lest they infect others). Despite the frustrations of dealing with new laws, the obsession to make things work kept Rafael busy and gave him purpose in an environment where he often missed his daughters, his home, and his friends. The laws in Colombia were cumbersome and constantly changing, but Rafael knew that he had a skill that was in high demand. Though he couldn't yet practice law in Bogotá, his training enabled him to figure out which rights Venezuelan migrants were entitled to. He also wanted to make sure people knew what they could expect and what they could not push for. There was little value in asserting rights when the other party was unwilling to give them.

Rafael's job, on a daily basis, was not only to tell people about their rights but also to teach them how to negotiate for them. For him the Venezuelans were his *people*, not his clients. *Client* was too formal a term and not a reflection of his relationship with them, a relationship that bordered on family. In his previous life in Venezuela, he'd never become emotionally invested in his cases. This was different. Success—when it happened—was a big relief. Failure was not only exhausting; it inflicted pain in ways he wasn't familiar with.

Rafael had learned that big announcements about refugee rights were more hype than substance. Often there was no formal law, and no real implementation. The announcements often caused confusion and misplaced excitement, which led to increased frustration and a sense of betrayal. Despite the breaking news about rights, the courts and the judges were still the same. The pace of the process was just as slow as before.

Over the last few months, Rafael had gotten quite comfortable understanding the text of what was already in the books and reading between the lines about what it may or may not mean. The real problem was in the implementation of these laws in an ever-changing country. Many of the Venezuelans who reached out to Rafael had already tried their luck at clinics or hospitals. They reached out to him after they'd been refused access or denied care at the last minute. Most had no legal standing, and for them there was little in terms of their rights to access care. There was the macro-law, which presumably applied to everyone, and then there was the micro-law, the one that mattered at the hospital or the clinic. It was this power dynamic, between two people separated by a barrier—one Colombian and one Venezuelan, one making decisions and one hoping for a miracle—that mattered. The micro-law had its own rules, which were driven by prior experience, xenophobia, momentary anger, or a flash of kindness. COVID-19 had added another level of urgency to this whole process, and now the denial of care, which wasn't at all unusual, could impact the health of other people who weren't sick to begin with.

In the midst of all this chaos, Rafael learned an important lesson—a lesson that a lawyer, who relies on the logic and order of the law, never really wants to acknowledge.

Rafael was part of several WhatsApp groups, some groups with participants living in Venezuela and some groups with participants living in the Venezuelan community in Colombia. Lately, he'd started noticing a trend. Some of the people he worked with were able to get care, even for relatively minor ailments, but others whose cases were much more severe and urgent couldn't get care. Initially, Rafael had thought that they were being helped by an NGO providing care through their clinics. That was sometimes true but not always. Sometimes certain people got care at a hospital or a clinic, while others were denied care in the same clinic. Both groups were undocumented.

Curious, Rafael inquired further. He questioned those who'd been able to successfully navigate the system, but they were guarded, almost secretive, about how they were able to receive care. Rafael persisted, using his goodwill capital within the community. Slowly he was able to piece together the puzzle.

The difference between those who were able to get care and those who weren't wasn't money (though Rafael suspected there may have been some bribes). Instead it was the *kindness of the hospital staff* combined with *a social network*. It was knowing which clinic to go to and when. Who worked at what time, and how kind that person was. There was an underground network of information, people, and places, which was allowing people to get the care they needed. Kindness of the locals was there, but not universal, you needed to know when and how to tap it. Beyond the laws and documents, there was another world where information was the most valuable commodity.

Henry requests medical supplies from a trusted doctor

As a result of Henry speaking with Dr. Julius about accessing medicines and COVID-19 tests, Dr. Julius later provided him with a few painkillers in shiny packets, which came from international charities. Henry graciously accepted them and thanked Dr. Julius for his kindness. But in reality, Henry knew these were of little use. While they could help one or two people in his flock, they were certainly not what he wanted for his brother's mental health or for protecting his people from COVID-19.

Henry felt a constant sense of anxiety. As long as he could remember, he liked to plan things and then organize himself and his actions according to that plan. He'd always been like this, adhering to a peculiar habit in his world where things remained unpredictable and where so much could change so fast. Yet, Henry always believed that his success in life was because of two things: his unshakeable Christian faith and his ability to organize himself. Lately, however, things were not going according to plan. He had hoped that with a few days left before his brother's arrival, he would be prepared. He and his family were going to downsize from two rooms to one. They would take the smaller room. Henry made sure that his brother got the best room in the house. But his brother's needs were more than just a room with a window that brought in fresh air in the morning. Solomon was ill and needed medicines and care, and Henry wasn't close to arranging that.

Things were shaky to start with, and then COVID-19—or as Henry liked to call it, "The Corona"—had completely upended his efforts.

It was not only Henry who was anxious and worried about a world turned upside down. His congregation was also confused and frustrated about what was going on. People in Henry's community had gotten used to the chaos of the war and had adapted to the uncertainties that came with it. This, however, was a new challenge and one they knew little about. The government was silent, and the people were picking up information from wherever they could: from friends in Sudan, family abroad, conversations among family, and bits of information that came from anywhere and everywhere. Members of his congregation were reaching out to Henry, as their pastor and as a medical professional, wanting him to tell them what may be happening now and in the near future. What should they do? What will happen to them?

An increase in infections came at a time when there was also an increase in violence in the country,[6] more than what had become commonplace. The conflict was not far from Malakan and it had affected livelihoods and the transport and movement of goods. The violence and the rise of COVID-19 infections meant that Henry had to worry about getting medicine not only for his brother's mental health but also to protect his congregation and family against COVID-19.

In this environment of desperation and frustration, there was, however, one resource left that Henry could still tap: Dr. James, an eye specialist Henry had known nearly all his life. Henry's father had known James's father, and the parallel acquaintances went back for generations. Henry knew that Dr. James wasn't a specialist in infectious diseases who could help with COVID-19 or a mental health specialist who could look after Henry's brother. But particular specializations mattered little at this time. What mattered more was that Dr. James had financial resources and a kind heart. He was from the same tribe as Henry, and he lived outside the country and, from what Henry had heard, was doing well in his practice. In a society desperately in need of cash and support, family ties and foreign currency mattered tremendously. Expertise in a particular area of medicine was much lower on the priority list.

James had left the country decades ago. He grew up in Wonduruba, but then moved to Uganda with his family to escape the violence of the first Sudanese civil war, which lasted from 1955 to 1972. He went to high school in Uganda and then to Kenya to study medicine. At that time, there was no medical school in the southern part of Sudan and, given the ethnic conflict, James applied to medical school at the University of Nairobi instead of the one in the northern part of Sudan. James was a brilliant student and had done well in high school. His brilliance and his passion for medicine was noted by others, and a Norwegian charity gave him a scholarship and supported his medical education. He finished his medical degree in Kenya and then stayed in Nairobi another two years for further training as an eye doctor.

Unlike most of his classmates, especially those who were not Kenyans, he didn't move north to the United States or Europe. At the time, the United Kingdom was a common destination for doctors from Africa. There was excessive racism prevalent in the clinical world in the United Kingdom but also a demand for foreign doctors. Many of James's peers chose to move to the United Kingdom despite excessive work, ill treatment, and massively unfair wages. James—now Dr. James—was different. He wasn't interested in building a life in the United Kingdom. He was instead driven by a passion to get Africa on its feet. He'd grown up at a time of hope and optimism for a fairer post-colonial world. He moved further south and landed in Zimbabwe in the summer of 1989. The newly independent nation was showing promising signs of social and economic progress, with a national growth rate among the highest in Africa during the 1980s.[7] This was a time when Robert Mugabe was still a hero, not just for Zimbabweans and Africans but for many in the West.[8] The country was eager to receive new talent from all over the world, particularly African professionals.

Dr. James did his post-graduate work in Harare, Zimbabwe, and then started working there as a doctor, first in a public hospital and then in private practice. He built his practice from the ground up. Over the years, his patients included not only Black Zimbabweans but also Germans, Austrians, South Africans, Indians, and of course hundreds of white Zimbabweans. He worked hard, did well, and developed a strong private practice. After two decades of working near the city, Dr. James moved to Mutare, a city in the highlands.

Mutare is beautiful throughout the year. In the spring the mountains change color with bright blossoms, and in the summer there are seasonal waterfalls throughout the landscape. The crisp winter air—Dr. James believed—would cleanse his lungs and his soul. This became his home. Using the savings from his practice, he bought land and built a hospital that provided free care for those who couldn't afford it. Soon he amassed a following among the locals, and the hospital continued to grow.

Though his parents had died and his siblings had moved out of Juba, and though Zimbabwe had been kind to Dr. James (he now had a wife and children), he didn't stop coming back to Sudan. For the first few years, he'd kept a low profile, coming in, helping some relatives and old neighbors, and then returning to Harare via Nairobi. From 2008 onwards, he came regularly to Juba and started a small practice with some friends at the hospital. Things changed rapidly after independence in 2011. Someone in the fragile government of the new nation found out about Dr. James, and his name started circulating as a possible administrator, even the minister of health. Dr. James was smart, successful, and fiercely patriotic. But he knew his limits. He met with local politicians and international agencies that were hugely influential in setting up the health care system in the new nation. The new government offered him the job of health minister. He considered it seriously, prayed about it, talked to his wife, and then declined. He simply couldn't trust the politicians who were in charge of all the affairs. He knew them all too well.

On one of his trips in South Sudan as he was ready to return to Zimbabwe, a relative asked Dr. James if he had time to meet a pastor from Malakan. Dr. James was a religious man and, despite his busy schedule in Juba, he agreed. The next day Henry showed up at his hotel in Juba.

Henry and Dr. James immediately bonded. They were from the same tribe and were about the same age. Their families had known each other, though the two of them had never met before. Since that meeting, Dr. James had helped Henry multiple times with cash and with medical supplies that he either brought himself or arranged through his contacts.

Henry recognized that Dr. James was resourceful but, with the crisis in Zimbabwe, things were getting harder for him as well. These were unusual times and Dr. James had always delivered. Henry contacted James through WhatsApp about his needs for his brother. James responded within a day.

Saida, at the legal clinic, hears of
a free mental health clinic for her brother

When Saida proposed to her brother the idea of going to the legal aid clinic, Tanvir showed little emotion. This was one of the lowest points in his life, and Saida had to make most decisions for him. On the day of the appointment, he didn't protest when Saida told him to come with her. He didn't say anything when it was time to go. Quietly, he walked alongside his sister on the roads, where potholes were now filled with trash and smoothed over by foot traffic.

Not far from their home, the legal clinic, the only one in the entire colony, was a busy place. The clinic consisted of four office rooms and a waiting room, which was full on the day Saida visited. Saida recognized some of the people waiting, and she exchanged pleasantries with them and asked about their families. They did the same.

She took a seat and Tanvir sat next to her. He was quiet and looked at the floor the entire time they waited. When their turn came, they went into one of the offices, a small place with sparse furniture. They sat on one side of a table, and on the other side sat a woman with glasses, a blue ballpoint pen in her hand, and a big notebook in front of her. She introduced herself. She was a lawyer and asked Saida the standard questions about her name, where she lived, where she was born, and why she was at the clinic.

Saida had prepared her answers in her head. She explained their situation of not having ID cards. She emphasized that the real reason she was there was to help her brother. It wasn't unusual for a woman to be deferential and suggest that the men in her family get their cards first. The lawyer had heard it many times before.

Throughout the meeting, Tanvir remained quiet, looking down and lost. The lawyer sensed that something wasn't quite right. She turned to Tanvir and asked him how he was doing.

Tanvir, initially quiet, slowly started to share. He didn't tell the lawyer anything about his abuse, but he talked about his severe sense of hopelessness regarding the system and his own life. He stopped mid-sentence and become quiet again. Saida wasn't sure where this was going. She was here to move things forward with their appeal for a CNIC (computerized national identity card[9]) not for the lawyer to talk to Tanvir about his struggles.

The lawyer took notes, asked for whatever documents Saida had, and then asked Tanvir to step out while she talked to Saida.

"I have a recommendation," the lawyer said.

Saida waited for the lawyer to finish her sentence. In this power dynamic, the only thing she could do was listen and not ask too many questions.

The lawyer told Saida that she recognized that Tanvir was struggling and suggested that Saida take him to a mental health clinic.

Saida explained that that was exactly what she wanted to do and was why she was there—first Tanvir needed a CNIC before getting mental health care in the public system. Saida felt she didn't need to remind the lawyer that they had no money for the private clinics. That part should have been obvious. She was confused as to where all this was headed. Saida told the lawyer that she needed a CNIC to get Tanvir examined.

"I know. But not all the clinics need CNICs," the lawyer said.

"The ones that don't require a CNIC require money."

"Not all of them," said the lawyer.

"What do you mean?" Saida was confused.

"Our parent organization runs a free mental health clinic for the community in Machar Colony, and I'll refer Tanvir to them right away. You can take him there next week."

Saida looked at the lawyer in disbelief.

Trusted networks include individual people, digital groups, and aid organizations

I have been conducting research in sub-Saharan Africa for well over a decade. A significant part of my research has focused on barriers to accessing health care commodities (medicines, diagnostics) and information among socioeconomically disadvantaged communities and vulnerable groups. It was one such trip that took me to Harare, the capital of Zimbabwe. Through some mutual friends and colleagues, I was introduced to Dr. James—the eye specialist in chapter 4 who helps Henry with medical supplies. Dr. James and I met at a hotel in downtown Harare. I had flown into the country from Nairobi, Kenya, a few days earlier. It was my first time to Zimbabwe, and I arrived largely unprepared for both the weather and the socioeconomic conditions. The electricity crisis that had been affecting the country for some time[10] had become so acute that our pilot had to land in near complete darkness. The entire airport was dark, with only a few lights on at the terminal. This absence of light followed me for some time. After I left immigration, I got a cab and rode through the city; I didn't see one light from the airport to downtown.

The day before I arrived, there had been yet another currency crisis along with the accompanying chaos, which included a kind of a run on the bank and general confusion about what the legal tender was in the country. As an outsider, unaccustomed to the situation and the changing policies, I was confused about how to pay for food and my taxi. Some merchants were accepting dollars in cash, others wanted payment through a credit card or a mobile money transfer. Some were not accepting anything except the bond note that had been issued by the government some time previously.[11] There was no defined exchange rate—inflation had reached a point that the numbers were no longer published.[12]

On the health front, the picture looked bleak. Medicines had become largely unavailable[13] or so expensive that they were generally inaccessible. With unemployment at an unprecedented level, stable income was a luxury for most people. Two days after my arrival, I asked some friends if I could speak to doctors who worked in the public sector. One friend recommended her own physician who worked at Harare Central Hospital, one of the largest medical complexes in the city. At the hospital, I met Dr. Ameer, a senior doctor, who had trained locally and had seen the ups and downs of the system. Dr. Ameer comes from a family of physicians: her father had been trained during colonial times and had seen the horrors of Zimbabwe's own version of apartheid. Dr. Ameer's family had plenty of deep scars to show from the evils of a brutal and racist regime.

"This is probably the worst I've ever seen," said Dr. Ameer. She was meeting with me and a group of six young doctors she was training. They all nodded in agreement.

However, the system, in its dysfunction, was still more functional than what I'd expected from reading the news and experiencing the chaos in the last few days. There was a brutal regime in power, inflation was off the charts, and little money was circulating. Robert Mugabe, the long-time authoritarian leader, was no longer in charge, after being unceremoniously removed,[14] but the new government seemed just as disconnected from the pain of ordinary citizens.[15] Why didn't the system collapse altogether?

The state was still absent when it came to health care and so were most of the international donors. International donors follow the political winds and often disengage (willingly or unwillingly) when the international politics of their rich country don't align with the local leaders. In the case of Zimbabwe, the late Mugabe years had *soured the mood in Europe and the United States, and international aid organizations and funding had all but dried up.*[16] *People were leaving the country in droves,*[17] *some going to nearby South Africa, where they were treated poorly and faced xenophobic attacks.*[18] *Others headed to Europe and the United States if they could find a way.*

I didn't want to be an alarmist, especially in the presence of the junior doctors, so I kept my questions to a minimum.

Afterwards, as Dr. Ameer and I walked to the large parking lot on a sunny and crisp July morning, I pressed her about what was really going on. I asked, "How do people survive?"

She smiled and said matter-of-factly, "It is Ubuntu.*"*

The term rang a bell and I asked her what it meant.

She explained that the term is broad and used across Africa in varying contexts, but for Zimbabweans, it means being connected to a deep human network and taking care of others.[19] *Whether it was pitching in, taking a loan, or selling items so that your family or community could get their medicines, people all across the country did their part to take care of others. This wasn't a favor to any-one but a* spirit *that ran through the community. This was par-ticularly true for Zimbabweans displaced because of poverty, violence in communities, or economic collapse. For community and family members living abroad,* Ubuntu *meant taking care of their loved ones, even if it involved back-breaking work.*

"Everybody is in it. This works like insurance based on the social network," explained Dr. Ameer.

| Survival Based on Social Networks

For those displaced in Zimbabwe, or for the poor and marginalized in any part of the world, *Ubuntu* or some kind of a "social network" of-fers a system that can be trusted. It's not a replacement for the public health system but rather it works in parallel and adds a layer of safety. When the public system doesn't work, this informal system of trust—a social network—acts as a lifeline.[20] It's not perfect nor comprehensive, but it can make a difference between life and death in case of an emergency.[21] The formation of networks of trust has been studied and debated by scholars. In practice, these structures are also flexible, and different aspects of the social network are tapped based on the severity of the need or the frequency of support that's needed. Accidents and a sudden deterioration of health is different from the frequent need for regular out-of-pocket expenses like buying monthly medicines. The network is just as important and central in preserving life as it is in taking care of funeral expenses at the end of life.

This kind of a social network is not limited to southern Africa, or Africa in general, nor is the value of a social network exclusive to financial support. The network offers reliable information, which can be just as valuable. Accessible and reliable information affects decisions and forms the basis of trust, which is a fundamental tenet of health care access among forcibly displaced communities. The social network among Palestinian and Syrian refugees in Beirut, Lebanon, is valuable in generating trust.

The families of many displaced Palestinians have lived in Beirut for over seven decades.[22] Among the Palestinian refugee camps, the Shatila camp (neighborhood) remains one of the most densely concentrated neighborhoods in the heart of Beirut,[23] not far from the glittering and exclusive penthouses in the high-rise buildings overlooking the Mediterranean. Young children seen today in Shatila are third- or fourth-generation Palestinians. This dense community, which started in 1949,[24] has continued to grow organically over the years as families have grown, but the space available to the refugees has shrunk. The intersecting electricity cables, water pipes, concrete blocks, and sewage lines[25] have created a unique, and increasingly dangerous, urban landscape. Electrocution is so common that those who die are referred to as "electricity martyrs."[26]

The Shatila camp was also a site of one of the worst massacres in September 1982, during the Lebanese civil war,[27] and the scars of that massacre are still present in the community. Then, when one would imagine there was no more space for people in this camp, the Syrian civil war broke out in 2011 (and is ongoing), and a third of the country was forced to flee, many to Lebanon. Some of these refugees were actually Palestinians who had first migrated during various conflicts in their homeland.[28] They'd found shelter (but not full citizenship rights) in Syria.[29] During the Syrian civil war, these groups returned to Lebanon. There were also Syrians among those who were displaced. Some are housed in many informal camps near the Syrian border, but these camps are viewed with suspicion by the displaced groups and offer little in terms of economic opportunity. There is an incentive to live outside the camps. Many of the twice-displaced Palestinians and many Syrians moved to Shatila,[30] and now live side-by-side with those who've lived there a long time.

The Palestinians living in Shatila prior to the Syrian civil war continue to have access to UNRWA clinics. These clinics, despite serious funding cuts, continue to provide a basic level of care. The clinics also employ a large number of Palestinians and provide a sense of trust and support. The Palestinians coming for care often know the staff. The Syrians, on the other hand, were (at least on paper) under the protection of UNHCR and not UNRWA[31] (because UNRWA's mandate does not cover non-Palestinians) and were becoming frustrated about inadequate services, lack of attention, and long queues.[32] In addition, discrimination issues were routinely reported.[33] However, as they moved away from the camps, many Syrians were no longer under UNHCR care. This was the same situation with the Syrian refugees who, for a variety of reasons, had never registered with UNHCR authorities to begin with or were in a perpetual state of ambiguous legal status, partly encouraged by the Lebanese state.[34] Many Syrians refugees moved to urban parts of Lebanon, including Shatila, and live in close proximity to the Palestinians.[35] Despite living side-by-side, both groups have their own networks that they rely on for medical advice and health care.

The Palestinians had been around for much longer, had developed their own network of trust, and were less suspicious of the Lebanese authorities. They were able to go to UNRWA clinics and pharmacies and sometimes to local Lebanese pharmacies where they knew the workers. The Syrians were the newcomers and experienced suspicion, hostility, and antagonism toward them. This environment created a sense of distrust among Syrians toward the authorities and impacted their choices in seeking health care. As a consequence of this distrust, they relied only on the network they trusted, even if this meant taking serious risks.

Syrian refugees in Beirut (and also in the camps) developed their own mechanisms to get their medicines from Syria.[36] This elaborate mechanism involved family members on both sides, taxi drivers who knew the routes well, and strategies to bring the medicines into the country. The fact that drugs were more expensive in Lebanon and that the Syrians[37] were not getting any subsidy made the choice easier. But it was not simply the economic argument working here. The Syrians didn't trust Lebanese brands and were much more familiar and comfortable with Syrian brands, which according to them worked much better.[38] Furthermore, the trust issue extended to who was selling the drugs. The pharmacist—who served as the de facto doctor, prescriber, and dispenser—could always be trusted in their hometown. Syrian refugees were more willing to accept the advice of the local pharmacist in their neighborhood, who would give them a good brand at a good price and would not cheat them, something that they could not say about the pharmacists working in Lebanese stores.

This aspect of the social network—risk and access to drugs—was not only present among the Syrians living in Shatila or other parts of Beirut. Those who were living in other camps were just as reliant on their own social network deep inside Syria to get medicines, along with associated information about which brands to take and which to avoid. Access to medicines, and health care, was more dependent on network than on proximity.

The trust factor also affects trust of institutions. Hospitals and clinics develop reputations for being hostile or welcoming, and within these institutions, there are people, wards, days, and times that are better than others. This information is passed through the social network. The network also has memory. The Palestinians in Lebanon avoid certain hospitals, not because of quality of care but because of discrimination and refusal to provide care.[39] Although the civil war ended decades ago, the memory and the social network continues to influence decisions about access to essential services including health care.[40]

| Information Gathering

Beyond financial support and trust, the social network plays a strong role in gathering and updating information about health care. It is the social network, more than the informational campaigns, that enables refugees and stateless people, who don't possess official documents, to find out where to go for health care.[41] As we have seen in previous chapters, those who have no form of ID in Pakistan's Machar Colony are formally excluded from accessing health care. The community is now aware, after a series of incidents, that appearing at a hospital is not without serious risks. It can mean more than simply the denial of care. It can also mean getting bullied, abused, or arrested by a police force that is known to abuse and harass them at will.[42] This is particularly true for women and girls, who are much more vulnerable to physical and sexual assault by police authorities or other law enforcement agencies. The risk of appearing at a hospital, without a clear plan, is therefore not insignificant. Yet, despite these challenges, the Bengalis of Machar Colony and other stateless groups from time to time must go to hospitals and seek health care. Risk mitigation is done through the memory of the social network based on prior experiences. The network's information core is updated through an organic mechanism of prior experience, word-of-mouth information, and digital social groups.

Several members of Machar Colony and local NGOs said they relied on word-of-mouth information and WhatsApp networks to guide the sick toward care.[43] Each successful episode further reaffirms the success of the network and strengthens belief in the power of the network. Each bad episode is also recorded in the collective memory of the network, eventually resulting in fewer people tapping into that resource. This is not to say that the network has perfect information, or that it's not prone to misinformation. Quite the contrary. It often has contradictory information, yet it continues to update itself over time.[44] There is no single curator or custodian of the network, nor is there a physical repository of information, only the beneficiaries of the network.

The informational core of the network provides portability and information that is relevant and contextual.[45] Migration journeys increase the risk of infection, injury, and disease. Ailments that are manageable at a single location become exacerbated due to travel, fatigue, and loss of access to trusted sources of care. Families (provided they have the means) often travel together and may include young children or pregnant women. Children who become malnourished and exhausted from the perilous journey can get seriously ill or even die. The demand is strong for quick and affordable health care along the route. Those who undertake such complex journeys are often unwilling to go to formal authorities, because of the risk of being incarcerated and deported or because of long lines and wait times. There is also the risk of becoming permanently separated from family. In these circumstances, the social network—through word of mouth, as well as through WhatsApp (and occasionally Facebook posts)—serves as an avenue to get care.[46] The memory of the network and the prior experience of others who have taken that particular route plays a role in risk mitigation. So does the source of information. Research has demonstrated strong reliance on Facebook and WhatsApp groups for health information by refugees coming from North Africa or Turkey into Europe.[47] This information ranges from buying medicines to accessing emergency services.[48]

The care provided comes in a variety of forms. In some cases, it is provided by small, grassroots NGOs or community-based organizations that have developed trust with other refugees and operate independently and are not formally part of the UN system or other large international aid agencies.[49] These groups or NGOs employ local staff and, due to their size, remain nimble and flexible. These agencies or groups do not demand extensive paperwork and registration documents. In other cases, the care is provided by other refugees who may have knowledge, resources, or medicines from their own visits. However, in most cases, this care is not for life-threatening (or otherwise serious) illnesses, and deals largely with ailments that don't require surgery, extensive and prolonged treatment, or hospitalization. In these cases of informal care, the most typical approach to treatment is through medicines, which are often available and used without any prescription, and shared with other community members.[50]

While the social network works for many, there are real risks and dangers associated with it.[51] First, there are questions about reliability.[52] Information shared may be outdated, and there may not be any actual services available, even when promised. With the rise in rumors and fake news, information can spread quickly without any verification. Patients desperate for help may therefore be misled and may not have any recourse in case of false promises. This leads to increased anxiety and a risk of furthering disease, as well as loss of money and essential time.

A second risk associated with these networks is that the quality of the information, products, and services is ad hoc. This has become particularly relevant during the COVID-19 pandemic.[53] In general, when it comes to social networks and social media, there is no supervision of the quality of products or services. WhatsApp messages or Facebook posts may be completely fabricated and can lead patients to providers who exploit their vulnerability. They may demand exorbitant sums or harass, assault, or blackmail patients.[54] Patients may also be exposed to counterfeit, substandard, or illegal substances provided in the guise of medical care. These products can increase the likelihood of severity of disease or mortality. They may also be ineffective, leading to a prolonged illness or development of complications, including drug resistance.

These networks, while beneficial for many, can also strengthen the black market of medical goods and services,[55] thereby creating both short- and long-term challenges for those who rely on them for health and well-being.

Chapter 5
Unregulated Medical Practices and Providers

Rafael is aware of the unregulated options for accessing health care in Bogotá

On the Simon Bolivar Bridge that connects Colombia and Venezuela, scores of vendors sell medicines to any willing customer.[1] Allergy medicines came in blue boxes, medicine for stroke in red, and medicine for heart ailments in white. The generic version of Tylenol, acetaminophen, was available in an aqua blue box. The city of Cúcuta, near the Colombian–Venezuelan border and one of the main entry points into Colombia for Venezuelans, was bustling with illegal pharmacies.[2] Some vendors worked on the street and were willing to negotiate the prices, while others had their own shops. There were plenty of makeshift pharmacies near hospitals as well. The ebb and flow of these pharmacies varied, based on how the Colombia government was feeling that particular month. Every time the government looked the other way, the number of street pharmacies increased. When the government cracked down, these pharmacies went underground, and the sellers switched their commodities. They abandoned pharmaceuticals and switched to what was in demand and not under the microscope that month.

Regardless of a particular commodity, the illicit trade has flourished in Cúcuta.[3] The market is flexible and sensitive to demand as well as the regulatory arm of the local government and the central government 500 kilometers to the south in Bogotá.

These informal markets, with a seemingly endless supply, provide drugs to Venezuelans patients. Among the biggest customers of this shadowy business are Venezuelan pregnant women who can't get care in Venezuela and come across the border on dirt roads to give birth at hospitals in Colombia.[4] Some would return after the birth, with boxes of medicines. Their medical needs went beyond just maternity services in the hospitals. They also needed medicines to prevent infection and control pain, and possibly get extra for others in the family. Underground networks of providers were happy to oblige them. But not every customer was a patient. Some were traders who would move the drugs back to Venezuela, buying them in Colombia[5] and contributing to the booming medical "flea markets." But it wasn't just Venezuelans who were selling at high markups. Colombians were happy to get in on the action as well. The trade was illicit and complex. Sometimes the lifesaving medicines that the Venezuelans bought into Colombia were originally meant for Venezuelans in Venezuela but had been smuggled across the border and then sold at a profit to Venezuelans in Colombia.[6]

Despite the presence of illegal pharmacies in Colombia,[7] the state has not given a clear, consistent response. The official position is that every drug needs a prescription, with the exception of over-the-counter medicines. Research, however, suggests otherwise. Drugs are easily available without prescription.[8] Rafael knew that too. With hospitals full or inaccessible to Venezuelans, and with the process of obtaining formal paperwork cumbersome and not guaranteed, it is a lot easier to just go to a pharmacy and pay in cash. Antibiotics are the most common drug requested and aren't hard to find. The market simultaneously operates both on the street and in the virtual world, and it flourished tremendously during the pandemic.[9] There are WhatsApp groups that connected buyers and sellers. A willing customer can also exchange medicines for food, or for other drugs, or for a promise of paying in the future.

Underground practices and the unregulated market don't only concern drugs, nor do they limit themselves to goods. There are medical procedures available for purchase. Underground abortion practice is an open secret.[10] Abortion is outlawed in Colombia, except in the case of abuse or danger to the life of the mother or baby. But the process of proving that was hard, cumbersome, long, and not equitable for the weak. Migration gave rise to the exploitation of women and girls, and prostitution was on the rise among vulnerable Venezuelans.[11]

Through his work with the Venezuelans who needed health care and support, Rafael had gotten to know young girls who were lured into prostitution, and met one who'd been working as a recruiter for her cousin's operation to find girls as young as fourteen. In addition to abuse and exploitation, there were also illegal abortions among Venezuelan women, including young girls, that led to infection, complications, and longer-term medical challenges.

Rafael also knew that others went to spiritual healers for treatment of their ailments. While the shamans and faith healers are more common in rural areas and in areas closer to the jungle, they found willing customers in Bogotá as well. In the southern part of the city, a particular faith healer had become especially popular for his miraculous treatments. Some Venezuelans who spoke to Rafael were too ashamed to admit going there; others found no contradiction in interacting simultaneously with doctors, underground peddlers, and shamans. They just wanted to stay alive. Shamans and faith healers were the last doors to knock on when all others were shut because of their poverty and then locked because of the laws in the country.

Henry sees an increase in the underground marketplace as refugees return

As people started returning to Malakan from Uganda, there was in-creased activity in the marketplace. Buying and selling that had be-come dormant, or perhaps had settled into a lackluster rhythm, was now starting to pick up. As people came back, exhausted from their journey, aiming to rebuild their homes, they needed supplies. People needed not only building materials, many of which were free, and tools, which were available on loan, but also medicines. More people in town meant more people who were sick—some from exposure to infection, some simply because of exhaustion from the journey. The small public health cen-ter in Malakan had closed due to lack of medicinal supplies, but the larger one in Wonduruba was still functioning. However, it wasn't al-ways well stocked. What was available in a particular month depended exclusively on the supplies coming in from Juba, and that chain was sub-ject to both conflict and corruption.

Henry had seen this demand for medicines being fulfilled by a series of providers, not just in Malakan but in all the other towns he'd been to while leading prayer groups with the regional bishop. There were some legitimate operations with real primary care clinics and real pharmacies. Most often, however, multipurpose shops doubled as pharmacies, despite having no staff trained in any relevant disci-pline. The supply chain for these stores was a bit dubious. Where and how they got their medicines wasn't clear, and Henry suspected that some of the medicines were meant to be given out for free and not sold. But he knew better than to question and disrupt what had become the norm.

Henry was well aware there was no regulatory system in place to check who was selling medicines and for how much. There wasn't a pre-scription system; people bought and sold based on their own judg-ment. Henry took some comfort in the fact that all drugs were imported, so they had presumably passed through the controls of international

NGOs. Hopefully this meant that there were few local knock-offs available. But NGO control meant that delays were common. When the NGOs waited for their own supplies, or when drugs were delayed from the point of entry to the markets in smaller towns, there was nothing on the shelves in places like Malakan.

People in Malakan had learned not to rely on NGOs. They looked for alternatives, and in Henry's town the only alternative came from ancient knowledge of herbal treatments. Passed down from one generation to the next, shared between the community, and free of cost, this was more reliable and equitable, although not always effective against complications. The efficacy of herbal medicines had been questioned during the HIV crisis,[12] and faith in herbal treatments (among some people) had eroded significantly. At the same time as international awareness shifted, plenty of HIV medicines and tests flooded health centers all over Africa. But that behavior was HIV-specific; little else changed in relation to other diseases. In Malakan now not everyone was HIV positive, and not every ailment was driven by the same virus. But in the vacuum that existed now, with not much coming through the roads from Juba, there was little else available. The choice to seek herbal remedies was partly based on history, partly based on necessity. The land—when not torched—was more reliable in providing treatments than offshore factories were.

Saida's camp system includes the use of untrained midwives, spiritual healers, and traditional practices

The legal clinic quickly got back to Saida. They suggested that Tanvir visit the mental health clinic near the legal clinic's building and run by the same organization.

Tanvir was suspicious. He considered Saida the only trustworthy person in the world, and he asked her what she thought. He'd become a person of very few words, but he asked if there was a catch. He was tired and didn't want another experience where his old wounds would be scratched raw. Saida was also puzzled about why anyone would want to care for someone like Tanvir. Weren't there more important things for them to worry about?

Saida, like everyone in the colony, knew that there was no real hospital in the colony, only two clinics, both recently built and both run by local NGOs. There used to be another one, run by MSF (Médecins Sans Frontières; Doctors without Borders), with a big sign, but they shut down their primary care operation in 2017[13] and started providing only specialized care for hepatitis. Saida was told they ran out of money for everything else. This sounded odd to Saida. How could they run out of money? They weren't doing any surgeries; the shelves barely had any medicines; and they didn't have a large staff. She'd always thought the people there worked not for the money but for the mission. As the doors to the MSF center shut, she realized she was wrong.

Like so many people around her, Saida herself had experienced a lack of basic medical care. When she was about to deliver her son, there was no nurse or doctor, no trained professional to take care of her. It was a young midwife, training on the job. Saida knew that no matter her condition during pregnancy, no public hospital in the largest and richest city in the country would see her. They would ask for a national ID card before anyone even examined her. A patient without papers was not a patient. To everyone, she was a Machar—a mosquito, a thing to be swatted away. There were private hospitals nearby and they wouldn't ask for an ID, but they'd ask for the other thing she didn't have: a hefty sum. No money, no doctor was how the system went for her. But she didn't complain because this was how it was for everyone around her.

During pregnancy, Saida was lucky. She didn't develop any complications and it progressed well. Those were among the best days of her married life. Her husband wasn't abusive during that period, and for the first and only time, he treated her with kindness. When the time came for delivery, the untrained midwife miraculously showed up at their house. Saida hadn't called for her, but people knew that Saida was pregnant and the midwives knew when to come. The social network operated on its own. Fortunately, her son was born without incident. Others in the community were less lucky. There were stories of women bleeding to death, babies born with permanent injuries, or both. Sometimes, if things got too complicated, the midwives gave up, even in the middle of the delivery. Such women were brought to one of the two clinics, not in an ambulance but in a wheelbarrow.

Lack of prenatal and delivery care was just one of the many signs of a vacuum in health services in the colony. In the absence of real care, the need was filled by people who claimed they possessed spiritual knowledge and ancient wisdom. These practices remained unregulated in the city.[14] Healers combined religion and spiritual practices with their techniques and prescriptions. Saida had been told by many that they had a solution to all of Tanvir's ills. Most of them were men, and in high demand. They enjoyed prestige and privilege. There were rumors that they were also quite rich, but they didn't show it. Everyone went to the shrines to pray and then to these healers before they went to see a medical professional. They operated from their homes and from the shrines, and every now and then there were reports of abuse of young girls and sometimes young boys.[15] But it was heresy to question their practices; people believed that even questioning their methods could bring God's wrath. Their ads were painted on the walls[16] and they remained above reproach.

Tanvir's case was further complicated by the general sense in the community that mental health wasn't a medical problem. It was a spiritual issue or a problem that needed to be fixed through prayer, and in some cases through force and discipline. Saida couldn't figure out why anyone would come to her colony and open a clinic for something that conflicted with the prevailing views. Yet, not everything made sense in the colony. The mental health clinic was an oddity here, and Saida was about to take her brother there.

Illegal practices and providers, traditional medicines, and untrained midwives

"We are not going to just sit here and die."

The sentiment, expressed by a Bengali community member in Pakistan, is a near-universal one among those who are unable to get medicines or treatment from their local public health system. What do people do when they are unable to access health care? No one gives up on life just because the state has given up on them. The instinct to protect young children or to knock on all doors to save a parent is innate and natural. But if most official doors are closed, which door does one knock on?

In many cases, the state looks the other way when care is needed but not always. The state, under pressure from its own citizens or in response to its own xenophobic impulse, may make it harder (or impossible) for disenfranchised people to seek health care through a clear, working system. The need of the patients, however, still remains. This need is often served by the black market, counterfeiters, illegal suppliers, and underground health care providers.

Tapping the intimate and broader social network sometimes leads to care and support and sometimes to increased risk and likelihood of an adverse outcome. The demand for care also emboldens and strengthens the black market. It is not only smugglers, in-country and en-route, who create the black market and who benefit from patients willing to risk their lives. Unqualified and unlicensed professionals, professing medical knowledge, also benefit from a similar situation.[17] The apathy of the local government, and neglect of patients in need, creates an enabling environment for unqualified medical practices to thrive. In some cases, the local government is a party and a beneficiary to this thriving illegal market.

Like human traffickers and smugglers, the black market and the unregulated medical practice sector thrive on demand. The provisions—qualified doctors, nurses, health professionals, medicines, medical devices—are in short supply. Qualified professionals have a limited incentive to work for free, unless it is through an NGO that itself depends on foreign funding to survive. There can also be a stigma associated with working for refugees, internally displaced persons, or the stateless—groups that may be viewed with suspicion by the society at large, including the clinicians themselves. This absence of available, qualified professionals further strengthens the underground activity of unregulated medical providers, who gladly fill the gap.

The black market for health care services and commodities is more like a market with several shades of gray. The customers are not only refugees, IDPs, and stateless persons but include the poor and the broadly marginalized, although the impact on the forcibly displaced is greater due to a combination of poverty, systemic exclusion, and lack of agency.

Healers and Midwives

Common unlicensed and unqualified medical services can be broadly classified into three categories including cultural/traditional medical practices provided by faith healers and midwives, illegal medical practices, and unregulated pharmacies and pharmaceutical practices. The first category of practices develops and thrives because of a belief and trust system. This includes traditional medical practices that are entrenched in the belief system of the patients and passed down from one generation to the next as part of culture and tradition.[18] Some of these practices are purely faith-based. In Karachi's Machar Colony, going to shrines of saints to pray for the recovery of a sick patient is quite common. It is also common in other parts of Pakistan, urban and rural, and among people who aren't stateless.[19] There are many charlatans and opportunists at these shrines who offer medical advice combined with spiritual practices,[20] but most of the advice given is of a benign nature and doesn't include any active intervention such as surgery, illicit pills, etc. The most common impact of these practices is that the condition of the patient worsens, and they seek help from other formal and informal sources.

The realm of faith also extends to traditional medicines, a practice entrenched in several cultures to varying degrees. For treatment, traditional medical practices often rely on herbal medicines and recipes that date back generations, sometimes centuries, although adulteration of herbal remedies with contraband substances is not uncommon and can cause serious health issues.[21] These practitioners often operate in the open without any serious threat of crackdown from the government. In some cases, traditional healers are highly sought after, even by the political elite, thereby giving them a sense of legitimacy and support.[22] These practices by faith healers are largely unregulated,[23] and most of their treatments do not require a medical license. In countries like Pakistan, homeopathic treatments fall in a similar category, where the practices are regulated by the practitioners' own professional organizations and not through the national medical regulatory system. The likelihood of falsified, substandard, and outright fake medicines in this domain is high.[24] The medicines, although widely available and sold in mainstream pharmacies, remain outside the purview of the national drug testing and regulatory structure.

Traditional structures that operate outside the formal health care system are not limited to diagnosis and prescribing remedies but also to providing services. The most common examples are the widespread practices of midwives and birth attendants during delivery.[25] Although midwives are certainly not limited to low-income settings, the presence of untrained midwives or birth attendants are more common in refugee camps,[26] and among those who can't afford a trained clinician, than they are in high-income countries.

There are global efforts to create a robust curriculum and oversight for midwives, and efforts are being made to bring midwives into national systems of training.[27] However, in low-income countries there is often little regulatory oversight.[28] Moreover, there are enough cracks in the system to allow for malpractice to continue. The lack of regulation and oversight allows for untrained midwives to operate and "learn on the job" from senior practitioners, who may or may not have had any formal training themselves. Some midwives are simply young daughters of existing midwives and are brought into the profession without any formal education.[29]

In Machar Colony, most mothers deliver at home with the help of a midwife or an untrained family member with prior experience, and several report harrowing instances at the hands of midwives. The lack of training in dealing with complications had resulted in excessive bleeding, loss of placenta, and other severe and permanent injuries. Maternal mortality due to preventable causes, and likely exacerbated due to unlicensed birth attendants, has also been reported in other communities.[30]

Poverty and difficult living conditions in rural communities, along with a lack of hygiene, can significantly increase the risk of infection and further complications.[31] Abuse (verbal, physical, and emotional) by unqualified and untrained midwives and birth attendants is well documented.[32] Issues of power dynamics cannot be ignored either.[33]

While the practices of traditional healers and midwives are not strictly underground, rarely are there any legal consequences for malpractice.[34] In engaging with healers, the patient and their family take on all the risk. Complications can result in injuries or scenarios that require urgent surgery or medical care, the absence of which leads to death or excessive morbidity. In some cases, these avoidable complications can lead to termination of pregnancy or inability to have children in the future. Stillbirths can lead to domestic abuse, abandonment, and/or divorce by the husband and permanent social stigma.[35] Despite these issues and the very real risks in engaging with unqualified and untrained midwives, they remain in high demand. Beyond tradition, another attractive aspect is that they don't cost as much as care at a private facility.[36] Also, these practitioners may be from the patient's community and sometimes might even work for free. Their ability to speak the same language and practice the same cultural, social, and religious norms is valued highly. The economics and the system of trust nudges the patient to seek them as the first point of support, instead of taking greater financial and security risks at the public or private hospitals and clinics or going to foreign midwives.[37]

Illegal Medical Practices

The second category of unlicensed practice is one that is truly underground, outlawed, and probably the riskiest in its potential consequences. The practices in this category are performed by unlicensed practitioners who claim to be legitimate doctors. Typically, it's well-known that they are unlicensed and have no formal training.[38] These practitioners don't claim to impart ancient wisdom and knowledge. Instead, they offer services that are typically offered in hospitals and clinics.[39] The evolution of their business varies around urban slums and refugee camps.[40] Quackery has also contributed to the rise of HIV infection in Pakistan in recent years.[41]

Often, these unlicensed practitioners offer a range of services, including surgery or orthopedic physical therapy or abortion services[42] in makeshift or underground clinics in unhygienic environments.[43] Such underground practices thrive in countries where abortion is outlawed or in places where the stigma of out-of-wedlock pregnancy is high.[44] These underground clinics—unlike herbal or traditional medical practices—are not advertised publicly; the information is passed by word of mouth and through the network of trustworthy friends. The clients are motivated less from a historical faith in their practices and more out of necessity, since the services are more complicated than simple medications. Here again, social stigma, lack of access, and cost play a role in creating a strong demand.[45] Young women in patriarchal societies often make up a significant part of the client base for these services.[46]

| Unregulated Pharmacies and Pharmaceutical Practices

The final group of providers is perhaps the most prevalent and widely accessed resource. It operates simultaneously in the regulated system and in the unregulated system, and offers mostly goods rather than services. Legitimate pharmacies that fill orders without requiring a prescription also fall in this category.[47] The pharmacy store is not in the shadows and serves both citizens and those without formal citizenship status. It operates on cash, and whoever can provide cash can be a customer. In some cases, the pharmacy is not a stand-alone business but part of a grocery and general merchandise store. Most pharmacy shops operate in a public space and don't need to hide their businesses from authorities (in contrast to the category of underground medical practices). However, not all the processes in these businesses are above board. For example, these pharmacies often employ people without any formal training in pharmacy,[48] despite the regulations and government requirements to have such training. These nontrained workers routinely provide medical counsel, prescribe medicines, and recommend doses.[49] They also give advice on which brands to use and which to avoid, and suggest medicines, such as carbapenems (an important class of antibiotics) or advanced steroids, which should only be taken in the most serious of instances.[50] In some cases, they are willing to inject a potent medicine into the arm of a willing patient.[51] The practice of dispensing and selling medicines without asking for a prescription, while widely practiced, is almost always against the public health guidelines of the country. The issue is not the law as it is written but its enforcement.

Because the pharmacy is able to provide a tangible product, and along with it, medical advice, the pharmacists (or workers) often become the most reliable and trusted source[52] for those who find clinics and hospitals closed to them. Because the pharmacy often employs local staff, social connections are either already present or are cultivated to ensure that the information accessed is reliable and up to date. Gaining access to drugs that should otherwise be reserved only for acute cases means that a connection with a pharmacist is a highly prized and valuable relationship.

Compared to the first two categories, the economic model is different in this third category. In the first two cases, the services are significantly cheaper than in the formal and regulated private sector. The services in the first two are also disconnected from any formal reporting mechanism, nor do they require paperwork typically needed in a public hospital. The case of pharmacies is different. For one, there are no special prices for refugees or the stateless (although in some cases there may be an elaborate credit system in place). Yet, there are attractive reasons to go to pharmacies. First, there is a strong element of trust, in both the person who works there and in the system. Pharmacies—unlike traditional medicine or underground practices—are connected to the formal medical system, which still serves as the gold standard among patients. It also builds confidence among the patients that they are being served by the same businesses and practices that other citizens are being served by.

Second, because the business model is based on products, not services, the level of risk is different. Third, pharmacy workers don't ask any questions about the buyer's origin country or citizenship status. By providing both advice (and in some cases a diagnosis based on visual symptoms or experience) and a product in a single visit, pharmacies are far more efficient than a clinic visit might be. Saving time and being efficient is valuable to those who understand they can be stuck waiting at a hospital or clinic, even when there's no cost for the service.

In Adjumani, in the northern part of Uganda for example, the clinics offer free service to any South Sudanese refugee. However, there's always a long line for a checkup, and the clinic pharmacist only fills the prescription after the patient has been seen by a doctor or nurse. This step-by-step service, in principle essential for quality control and appropriate dispensing of drugs, means long waits for the patient, often in scorching heat without any shade or in packed rooms with no ventilation. It's not unusual for a patient to return the next day or day after to finish their visit.

Only a five minutes' walk from the free camp clinic is a pharmacy where plenty of drugs are available. The person dispensing the drugs is not a pharmacist but seems to exude confidence and provides information about diseases, does a visual inspection of the patient, and hands out the drug in a matter of minutes. There's no paperwork required, no forms stating prior medical history or citizen status. Most transactions are based on cash, but the shop also extends credit, based on prior history and the relationship between pharmacist and customer. Even though a customer can get medicines for free at the clinic, business is always booming at the shop. Many customers are willing to forgo the free drug and pay the moderate price, demonstrating that they value their time and hassle-free health care.

Access to drugs is also not always through regular pharmacies. Unregulated vendors who sell drugs on the street routinely appear under certain circumstances.[53] The presence and capacity of these street vendors depends on both the willingness of the government to tolerate the illicit businesses and the strength of the networks that smuggle drugs. During the peak of the economic crisis in Zimbabwe, informal markets would often appear and thrive in Mbarre,[54] where prescription-only drugs would be easily available. Historically, Zimbabwean pharmacies required a prescription to dispense drugs,[55] but as the state collapsed from within due to economic turmoil, corruption, and nepotism, access to drugs became tenuous and gave way to an informal and unregulated pharmaceutical sector.[56]

A similar situation was seen in Colombia where, historically, prescription laws were largely enforced. However, as the Venezuelan crisis escalated, medicines became available outside of tightly regulated pharmacies in Cúcuta and other border towns.[57] The presence or absence of these unregulated vendors correlated with a government crackdown and also with the number of migrants crossing. For example, as the number of migrants increased, the burden on the formal sector also increased and the ability of regulated clinics to serve everyone decreased. Then the informal sector would thrive, offering solutions to those who didn't want to be at the back of the queue. The government was more tolerant of the informal sector at that time. At other times, when the migration rate slowed, the informal sector faced harsher crackdowns from the government.

Pharmacies can offer a wide range of products for the same ailment. Some drugs may be imported, and others may come from local or regional manufacturers. There may be drugs sold that are completely counterfeited.[58] Their quality may or may not be known to the pharmacists. The presence of various brands (and sometimes varying quality) allows vulnerable people to access drugs based on their purchasing capacity.

For those who may be crossing international borders on complicated multi-country routes (e.g., from Afghanistan via Iran and Turkey into Europe), the presence of pharmacies that do not require a prescription can offer a lifeline. Antibiotics and other anti-infectives can make a difference between life and death, especially given the high likelihood of infection during a journey that includes experiencing close contact with various people, living in tight spaces, and taking in limited nutrition.[59] For people entering a country without a formal visa, the only chance of fighting disease is through accessible drugs; therefore drugs that can be purchased without a prescription can make a big difference in their lives. Just as the use of antibiotics can fight life-threatening infection, overuse or abuse of antibiotics is also the driver of long-term and possibly deadly antibiotic resistance.[60] The battle between excess and access plays out in full force in the lives of forced migrants.

Chapter 6
Accessing Health Care
via Digital Technologies

Rafael's WhatsApp messages typically arrived throughout the day, but it was the evening when his screen would light up nonstop with new messages and urgent requests. Rafael wasn't certain why most people contacted him in the evening, but he thought it was because internet connectivity was better in the evening or because the people who contacted him were done working for the day and were now able to get near a Wi-Fi spot. WhatsApp was an invisible thread that tethered Rafael to the Venezuelans in Bogotá and beyond. It wasn't just him, but everyone he knew relied on WhatsApp for most of their communication. What would have happened ten years ago, Rafael often wondered. He'd heard that, in some places, Facebook was also used to share information among groups, but Rafael's experience was different—only WhatsApp was used. People not only made requests via WhatsApp but also shared information and documents. It was also how rumors circulated about the better doctor, the kinder nurse, and the evil administrator.

Rafael knew he wasn't the only one dispensing legal advice via Whats-App. His Venezuelan friends had told him that they could also get medical advice from doctors using WhatsApp. The Venezuelan doctors, both in the country and outside, were able to meet with uninsured Venezuelans via WhatsApp and offer their diagnosis and advice. It wasn't unusual for Venezuelan doctors to work in Colombia, and many were familiar with the system and its oddities. Venezuelan doctors, more than other nationalities, had long had an easier route to practice in Colombia. It was part of a scheme between Colombia and its neighbors that allowed the recognition of medical degrees and the possibility to practice among neighboring countries. Colombian doctors had long felt that Venezuelan medical training was inferior, but it had never been an issue until the Venezuelan crisis. Before the crisis, there were plenty of openings, particularly in smaller towns, where Venezuelans filled the demand. But now there were concerns that Venezuelan doctors were giving advice to Venezuelans that wasn't accurate or up to date. Some hospital administrators worried that Venezuelan doctors were mentoring their compatriots on how to circumvent the system.

Rafael was dismissive and unconcerned about the feelings of Colombian doctors. It was better that patients were getting advice from doctors rather than from shamans and frauds.

Henry's privilege: Owning a smartphone in South Sudan

Henry was the only person he knew in Malakan who had a smartphone. He'd gotten his Chinese-made phone two years ago in Juba. He had to save money for several months before he could buy it. It wasn't that no one in Malakan knew what a smartphone was or knew that some people like Henry had one; it was simply that phones were too expensive for most people. And there was no one in Wonduruba who sold phones. You had to go to Juba to get one, at a shop that only sold and repaired phones.

Getting the phone was only one part; having a cell tower nearby was another. About a decade prior, when the situation in the country had improved, albeit briefly, new cell towers were installed throughout the countryside. Academics and entrepreneurs, and those in the business of projections, were constantly talking about cell phones reaching everyone, and how the African economy would leapfrog forward in areas including digital banking, information, and health care. The euphoria also reached South Sudan. Juba was first to get connectivity through cell towers, but it wasn't long before Wonduruba and then Malakan also got cell towers. Used and refurbished cell phones penetrated the market, along with phone plans. Some people in Wonduruba also received special training in fixing old and broken phones. In the absence of reliable grid power, there were new ideas about charging phones using solar power.

But it was all short lived. Conflict caught up with the towns, up and down the country; and while smart phones became more common in places like Juba, places like Malakan and Wonduruba went in the other direction. Many cell towers in the entire region of Central Equatoria were destroyed.[1] Henry doesn't recall when it happened, or whether it was intentional or not, although he has his suspicions about which group specifically targeted the towers. The towers were destroyed years ago and never rebuilt. Henry thinks they are likely to stay like this for the foreseeable future. Working cell towers are no longer a priority.

In Henry's hometown, mobile phones play no role in seeking or accessing health care. Information travels through word of mouth in the tightly knit community, not through WhatsApp. Many have never heard of WhatsApp. Technology beyond cell phones is just as unreliable and unpredictable. Diagnostic tests for malaria and HIV are numerous, and often in surplus, but COVID-19 vaccines are nowhere to be found.

Life goes on, with or without technology.

Saida avoids digital registration

For the first appointment, Saida took Tanvir to the mental health clinic. A young woman, who worked at reception, received them. She asked

Saida the same standard questions she'd answered at the legal clinic. The young woman then politely asked Saida to wait outside while the therapist spoke to Tanvir. For forty-five minutes, Saida waited outside. She'd never been to a mental health clinic, so was unsure what might have been going on inside. She felt a sense of anxiety, anticipation, fear, and hope.

Finally, Tanvir emerged. Although the change in him was small and perhaps not observable to others, he seemed more positive to Saida than in the past. As they walked home, he spoke more than usual. When they reached home, he told Saida that for next week's appointment, he would go himself. Saida didn't have to accompany him anymore. That moment, with tears in her eyes, Saida felt happier than she had in years.

Just as Tanvir's life was taking a turn for the better, the COVID-19 pandemic struck the country. First, there was denial[2] across several regions and socioeconomic sectors in Pakistan. No one believed that deaths in the colony were due to a new disease coming from outside the country. People were always sick in the colony, and everyone said that life and death were in God's hands anyway. Old people got ill and died. Sometimes young people did as well. This is how life worked in the colony. You didn't need announcements from the ministries and health departments to tell anyone that.

Plus, there was no way to know whether anyone had caught the disease or not. Who was to say that there was a new disease among them? Yes, there were tests, but they were expensive, costing as much as a month's salary for the shrimp peelers in the colony. Why would anyone want to get tested and spend their entire salary on it? And if you did get tested and it was positive, then what? A better option was to seek care in the colony with the healers who knew how to treat everything with their special chants and prayers. Whether or not there were tests available in the market didn't matter; they weren't for people like Saida.

That was in the beginning of the pandemic. But over the course of a few months, the mood in the colony started to change. Even without anyone actually counting, people realized there were more deaths than normal. People who weren't chronically ill were dying as well. The explanation that Saida heard was that COVID-19 may or may not be a real disease, but it was a conspiracy to target Muslims.[3] Saida personally knew people who had gotten ill, people who had a fever, chest pains, and severe breathing issues. And if they recovered, the recovery was slow, and they weren't quite the same. But there wasn't much they could do. Except keep quiet and not tell anyone.

Life went on in her neighborhood but with greater anxiety. Tanvir was getting better, but everyone else was nervous. Saida was worried about people in her home: her son, who spent most of the day playing outside; her brother, who was struggling; and her mother, who was old.

One day, she heard from a neighbor that in Karachi there was available a *teeka* (the local word for a vaccine or a shot), but it was only for those who were connected: ministers, politicians, army officers, businessmen, and others in their networks. Not people like Saida.

Saida then heard that the country had run out of vaccines.[4] She assumed that all the "important" people had used up all the stocks. A few weeks later there was another vaccine in the market, supposedly from Russia. It was made available at an upscale hospital for 50,000 Pakistani rupees. This was more than Saida could earn in six months.

The same neighbor who told Saida about the vaccine said it was a blessing that there was no vaccine for them. The neighbor had seen a video on her phone, sent to her via WhatsApp, and she was adamant that it was true. The video showed that the vaccine was going to mess with young women's fertility.[5] Without a husband around, this was the least of Saida's worries. Then she was told by another friend that the vaccine was another conspiracy, and it contained microchips. The last straw was the video Saida saw herself on her neighbor's phone where a serious-looking person, who was known to be a holy man of great virtue, said that everyone who would got the vaccine would die within two years

Another wave of the disease came, and more people got sick. More people died and were buried quietly since no one wanted to talk about the disease. Around the same time, Saida heard that there were more doses of vaccine available in the country. People like Saida now had a chance. She convinced her mother that they should get the vaccine. She was also concerned for her brother, but maybe he could wait. She asked around if there was a way to get the vaccine, since she'd heard that it was free and available. It was free, she was told, but not for her.

"Why not?" she asked.

"Do you have a CNIC?"

"No."

The person she asked didn't have to reinforce his point.

CNIC. The same elusive card that Tanvir needed to get care. It had become a gateway to their health care. A key to stay alive. A key that Saida didn't have. She'd attended school for only a few years. She'd learned to read but she wasn't conversant in English. She didn't know what *CNIC* stood for, or that it was an acronym, with the *C* standing for "computerized," a salute to the modernization campaign in Pakistan. She didn't know that the computerization of the national ID system was hailed as a watershed moment in the country, a celebration that Pakistan was now proudly in league with advanced countries. But she did know that ever since there was a new system, one that relied on computers, her family had been formally kicked out of the folds of society. This isn't how it had always been. Both her father and mother possessed documentation that they showed to get by in the past. But starting in 2000, as the country moved to a computerized system, she was formally stateless. An outsider.[6]

The government, through their computerization of ID cards, had even tried to formalize her outsider status. In the past fifteen years, several campaigns were launched to get Saida and her family and others like them to register as aliens in the country. To permanently declare them as noncitizens. This move had created severe anxiety among the members of the colony. There was resistance to register as aliens, but the government had pushed hard. Many were coerced, tricked, and harassed to give their biometric data and receive a permanent status as those who don't belong. Those who registered would get a card, called a NARA (National Alien Registration Authority) card, a certificate of unbelonging.

Trust in the government was at an all-time low. Even the word *biometric* sent chills down the spine of members in the colony. Saida and her family had resisted and so far had been able to stay away from the NARA system. Saida had been advised, by people in the same legal clinic that helped her with Tanvir, never to give her biometrics, never to agree to sign a form.

The COVID-19 vaccination campaign changed again in spring and summer of 2021.[7] Under pressure from human rights campaigners and epidemiologists who wanted everyone to get vaccinated, the government softened its stance. Anyone, whether or not they were formally citizens, could get their first and the second doses. Saida seemed relieved. She asked if her mother could get the vaccine.

"You need a CNIC," she was told.

"We don't have one," she said quietly.

"Okay. You need to have a mobile phone in your name."

Saida didn't have that either. A mobile phone required a SIM card, and a SIM card required a CNIC.

"Do you know anyone who has a phone? You can give their number."

Saida knew people who, through their connections and social network, had gotten a mobile phone. She could give their number. She was determined to get her mother the vaccine.

She was disappointed to hear that the vaccination site was a forty-five-minute taxi ride from her home, and twice as long by bus. But she could manage that. As she was about to go home and tell her mother about the appointment, she asked one more time to confirm.

"So, nothing else is needed from our end, right?"

"No, nothing else. Just have someone's phone number available."

Saida nodded.

"There will be a line, and your mother will get her shot after she is fingerprinted and her biometrics are recorded."

The dreaded word again. Saida was no longer sure if her mother would ever get a shot.

Digital technologies can be a lifeline but can also be weaponized

A *smartphone is a lifeline for the refugees and the forcibly displaced*. This message is not only about a smartphone being a *proverbial* lifeline but a *literal* one.[8] The loudest voices proclaiming this are researchers and those who work at international agencies. Some argue that smartphones are more important than health care access or housing.[9] But just because there's a chorus of voices singing the same tune, is this message true, or universal? Is technology the great equalizer, the path to the promised land of equity? Or is it simply a tool that creates inequity and, in some cases, even greater risks for forcibly displaced communities?

A smartphone is less of a device that works like a phone and more of a resource that provides information that can save lives.[10] Apps are no longer just a way to connect with loved ones, or see photographs of friends, but are used more and more as a source of real, contextual, and tangible information. These apps—from the perspective of those who are forcibly displaced—can provide them with not only lifesaving information about transportation routes and checkpoints but also specific information about medical treatment. Internet connectivity is globally increasing, and data plans are now much cheaper than previously. A smartphone has become an essential commodity, one that is both prized and protected by those on the move.[11] However, smartphone usage is certainly not universal, and those who are on the lowest end of the poverty spectrum do not have access.[12] There is a gendered dimension as well, with fewer women than men owning a smartphone.[13] Yet, there is a marked increase in the global smartphone usage among low- and middle-income countries.[14] The used phone market has brought in millions of people—including refugees, migrants, and stateless communities—to tap into real and virtual networks.[15]

While the Facebook app continues to be a tool to organize (and at times undermine democracy and legitimize hate), another product owned by Meta Platforms (formerly Facebook)—WhatsApp—has become increasingly popular among migrants, refugees, and stateless communities.[16] WhatsApp messages and chat groups allows them to learn who may be able to give them medicine to heal their child when the public system denies them care.[17]

For groups on the move between countries and borders, WhatsApp groups also provide archival knowledge, based on prior experiences of others who have traveled the same path.[18] The bandwidth required for WhatsApp is relatively modest and becoming more accessible, and hence the messages are easier to transmit and receive. In many ways, WhatsApp access shapes the map of the journey, allowing people on the move to avoid certain hospitals and clinics while prioritizing others. The voice message feature, in particular, comes in handy, making it possible for those who might not know how to read or write or may be unfamiliar with the script on the phone's keyboard. An essential feature of seeking health care is trust, and the social network and smartphones have enabled people to tap into that trust, memory, and network capital.

Digital Technologies and Aid Delivery: Not as Easy as It Sounds

The rise of digital technology, associated affordability, and access has created a new space where many have gathered, in addition to refugees, migrants, and stateless persons. Large international aid agencies and institutions also embrace widespread use of digital technology.[19] There is a lot of interest, investment, and excitement about computing, artificial intelligence, and data.[20] Some of it, unfortunately, is more hype than substance.[21]

The claim by international agencies, at least on paper, is that digital technologies will build in much needed efficiency in the system of aid delivery. These technologies will tackle corruption, reduce waste and redundancy, and cut out intermediaries and cumbersome bureaucratic processes. International agencies also claim that technologies can offer a fairer system, and people who have been getting more than their fair share from the already-shrinking pot of resources would not be able to take away anyone else's share. By extension, the argument goes, those who are often unable to get their fair share—for example, women, or those with disabilities, or those who are lower in the camp hierarchy— will now have an equal opportunity to receive aid.

But the reality is more complicated than the big claims. For instance, in early 2016, the UNHCR introduced a biometric identification system that scans a user's iris pattern in the Azraq refugee camp in Jordan, to be used with Syrian refugees to streamline shopping for essential items such as food, oil, bread, soap, etc.[22] There was a lot of fanfare about new technology coming to the camps to provide food assistance. The program was designed to create cashless transactions, using the iris scan as ID. To shop, refugees had to stand in front of a camera that was installed in the market. The technology inside the camera would then recognize the person who was enrolled, and then they could shop. The system kept track of expenses, and the refugees didn't have to pay in cash for the objects that they purchased. While dubbed a major advancement in creating efficiency and decreasing the burden on the refugee to keep cash, cards, or documents, the program failed to get everyone excited.

A number of refugees enrolled in the system said that they were never told that the program was optional, and no information about opting-out was provided. This issue of messaging, consent, and clarity about technology has come up in several other instances as well. Adding to that, the experience of getting their iris scanned was unusual and seemed intrusive to the refugees. The iris scan ID was only collected for the head of the household, not for every member. This posed several practical problems. If the head of the household was unable to go to the supermarket (if, for example, they were tired, unavailable, or pregnant), no one else could shop in their place. If the mother was the designated head of the household, she would have to bring all her children to the store. These situations created a rush at the store, and disincentivized those who were ill, pregnant, or worried about the chaos at the market. Designed to increase efficiency of the system, and decrease the hassle of IDs, the iris scan ended up creating another hassle for the refugees. The iris scan program, despite the initial excitement, hasn't been rolled out widely in other camps outside Jordan.

The iris scan project also highlighted another, and perhaps bigger, challenge with using digital technologies: privacy and data protection.[23] There is no clear international law that governs privacy of biometric information of refugees. International agencies are working with a patchwork of regulations, most of which are not enforceable in communities that are denied political, social, and financial agency. Transparency in communication to the refugees about their rights creates further problems.[24] There is often no quality control in exercising how the information has been provided, whether that information is accurate and up to date, and how well it has been conveyed. In addition, with communities on the move, a single country regulation is not adequate.

In the case of a breach of privacy, however, refugees have little recourse.[25] They are often unaware that their data has been compromised, and due to persecution, fear, and anxiety about the future, they are often unwilling or unable to pursue legal action against anyone. They are also often unaware of their rights, and many have no contact with lawyers. With courts not prioritizing refugee rights in many countries, lack of clear policies about who would be held responsible for any data security breaches, and confusion about which court would have the jurisdiction to hear such a case, there is a lot that remains to be done in data protection and privacy of vulnerable groups.[26] Holding an international agency responsible for its bad data security policies is unlikely to become a high priority in a climate of xenophobia and one where people on the margins have a deep sense of anxiety and depend significantly on international aid.

The privacy issue is not just a theoretical or an abstract question; it is one that has real implications for the safety, livelihood, and well-being of refugees. In 2021, Human Rights Watch (HRW) reported that the UNHCR had been collecting biometric data from Rohingya refugees living in camps in Bangladesh, after fleeing Myanmar.[27] The biometric information, collected during registration for aid cards, was then shared with the government of Bangladesh (without informed consent), who in turn shared it with the government of Myanmar, the very state that had been carrying out ethnic cleansing against the Rohingya. Sharing this information undoubtedly put the Rohingya at risk[28] and affected their ability to return to their country. It could also put them at a disadvantage for any future employment or access to education or health services.

Data storage has become cheaper and easier, and now it can be stored for years or decades. A state that chooses to use that data can therefore make an impact not only on the individual but also on the extended social network. Guilt by family association continues to impact communities for generations.

How did the data end up getting shared with the government of Myanmar? What was the role of the UNHCR? The answers remain murky. This situation highlights the need for transparency and underscores the inherent risks of new digital technological solutions. The Rohingya refugees who were interviewed by HRW said that they were not told how the data (e.g., analog photographs, thumbprint images, and other biographic data) would be used. They were only told that it would allow them to get the smart card to access essential aid. After registering for the biometric system, they were given a receipt in English (a language that most Rohingya do not speak or read). That receipt included a question (in English) asking if the data could be shared with the government of Myanmar; the box was already checked as "yes."

The UNHCR staff defended their approach and said that in each case the refugee consented to their data being shared. Nearly all the refugees interviewed by HRW disputed this claim. One refugee, who did acknowledge his consent, pointed to a bigger problem: an asymmetrical power relationship. "I could not say no because I needed the Smart

Card and I did not think that I could say no to the data-sharing question and still get the card."[29]

Questions about the meaning of informed consent in these circumstances remain poorly understood.[30] Policies of ethics in data collection are often cut and pasted from other instances, without a recognition of the local challenges, context, and power dynamics at play. Despite repeated instances of miscommunication and misunderstanding, the problems of informed consent persist in sharing personal biometric data of the forcibly displaced.[31] This is due in part to a top-down approach from host governments and international agencies willing to go along with minimal engagement from refugees or refugee support groups. In addition, digital technologies are not codeveloped with refugee support groups. Refugees, instead, are treated simply as recipients of such technologies (with the assumption that whatever is developed is good for them) without real ways to opt out.

Researchers point out that there is also an inherent hypocrisy when it comes to protecting refugee data. Zara Rahman, a journalist who reported on the Rohingya data breach story, has argued, "There is no way that the personal data of nearly a million European people would be treated like this without a massive outcry, without resignations and policy overhauls, without fines, firings, and legal ramifications."[32] Yet, none of this has happened. The outcry about refugee data protection died out quickly weeks after the HRW report.

The idea of "smart" ID cards is being tried in other countries as well, from Pakistan[33] to the Dominican Republic.[34] While they seem to be popular among the general public (i.e., not forcibly displaced persons) and presumably have improved processes, such as passport applications, and access to health cards, they are also powerful tools that can be weaponized to deny communities their basic rights.

In Pakistan, among the Bengali population, the issue of computerized national identity cards (CNICs) is a particularly sensitive topic. A computerized system is able to connect entire families together in a single database, and investigating a single member can impact the ID cards of the entire extended family. Bengalis who are viewed with suspicion, or who may not have all the necessary documents, are denied a CNIC and, as a consequence, their entire family may lose privileges (due to blocking the card of a single person in the larger family circle). This results in denial of essential and, at times, life-saving health care services. During the COVID-19 pandemic, the government for months required that each citizen must have a CNIC in order to get vaccinated.[35] Their argument was that vaccine doses were limited and could not be wasted. The only way to track who was vaccinated (and who can therefore get a vaccination certificate) was by tracking their CNIC. In the absence of that, the stateless population, despite being interested in getting a vaccine, were denied access.

This policy was eventually changed in late spring and early summer of 2021,[36] when the government said that if someone didn't have a CNIC, they could use other forms of identification or a smartphone. Unfortunately, getting a smartphone is not easy if you don't have a CNIC. Furthermore, the vaccination centers that were willing to accept other forms of documentation were often located too far from the homes of the stateless Bengali population in Machar Colony. Government officials were then able to use their preexisting narrative: the government was doing everything it could to provide care, but the Bengalis were unwilling to do anything to change their own situation.

Digital Technology Can Lead to a False Sense of Progress

The issue with vaccines is the latest in a long line of exclusionary policies in Pakistan. The stateless Bengali population was forced and coerced to register as aliens in 2000 through a program called National Alien Registration Authority (NARA).[37] The controversial program created trauma and anxiety among the Bengalis because registration meant forfeiting any right to citizenship, including birthright citizenship. However, there were few options: they could either register or face jail. Many resisted, and the program was abandoned in 2015 only to reemerge with new promotional videos in 2021.[38]

145

Digitization can also take away citizenship, and consequently access to public health facilities can be quickly curtailed. Countries may choose to exclude from its citizenry a certain group of people (e.g., Haitian-descended citizens in the Dominican Republic).[39] This can lead to devastating consequences for communities that are already marginalized. The digital technology boom that has penetrated the humanitarian sector and has often been presented as a democratic and a fair approach, can in fact push out much further those who are already on the fringes. It can also give states near-complete power over the lives of vulnerable communities and their complete identity, while giving few options to those who are deprived of any political, social, or financial agency.

Regarding access to health care in low- and middle-income countries, digital technology has been hailed as a big boost and an opportunity to increase access, decrease bureaucratic burden, cut waste, and improve patient experience.[40] There are, however, several problems with this sense of euphoria. First, technological solutions work *within a system* and are not a substitute for robust primary care. Alain Nteff, a technology entrepreneur from Cameroon, says that a smartphone is no substitute for a midwife.[41] The reliance on technology, particularly mobile technology in the domain of health care, has created a false sense of progress. Not only do these technologies act as a poor bandage, they also enforce financial and socioeconomic inequity. The poorest communities, in both rich countries and low-resourced countries, are therefore left out of a health system that relies heavily on access to a product that is not cheap or provided equitably by the state.[42]

While refugees, migrants, and stateless persons may rely on WhatsApp and Facebook, the impact remains uncertain beyond information sharing and creating a real change in their health indicators. The impact of technology beyond apps is even weaker. In matters of health, digital technologies get a disproportionate share of coverage and attention. Yet, from diagnosis to treatment, from disease management to long-term care, digital technologies cover only a fraction of the overall technological landscape.[43] Diagnostics, vaccines, pharmaceuticals, prosthetics, and other technologies are all part of the technology land-scape. These devices and systems are just as essential for diagnosis and treatment, and can't be converted into an app. In fact, beyond digital technologies, technological innovation (from the development of new therapeutics to new diagnostics) has remained largely out of reach for refugees.[44] In this case, the painfully slow trickle-down effect has largely been at play. There are some efforts to create 3D-printed prosthetics[45] and diagnostics, but they haven't reached any appreciable level of success and are far from accessible to refugees and stateless persons.

Technologies Are Rarely Developed Specifically for the Poor

Technologies developed specifically, and exclusively, for refugees, forc-ibly displaced persons, and the stateless are extremely rare to the point of nonexistent.[46] There are several reasons for this. The first and most prominent one is the lack of funds available to develop novel and purpose-built technologies to address the complex health needs of the forcibly displaced.[47] While scientists often describe their work as the quest for knowledge, driven by curiosity, technology development and dissemination requires business models that go beyond good intentions. Any development process considers the real costs and accounts for fail-ure. Clinical trials—at least ones that meet ethical standards—are ex-pensive and contain many steps that can take years. Similarly, develop-ment demands quality control that requires infusion of significant financial resources. In a typical innovation business model, these costs are recovered by the innovator, or their financial backers, through prof-its and eventual payment for goods and services. Money made by sell-ing the product to the final customer, be it an individual, institution, or state, is fed into the business model as a consideration about whether to move forward with development or not.

The lack of capacity to pay by refugees as well as by institutions working for refugees (which itself is dependent on NGOs, foreign aid, or charity) means that there are no real resources available to develop technologies for that market. Issues related to patents and intellectual property are also important. In many cases, the patents may not hold up or be recognized in countries where the technologies are implemented. The lack of protection of intellectual property can deter potential innovators and investors. Upfront costs to apply for patents can also be significant, and recouping those costs is not guaranteed.

The second reason that technologies are rarely developed specifically for refugees is that incentives from host countries, where refugees and stateless persons reside, are few. In many cases, the refugees and stateless are viewed as a security risk, and hence local host countries don't want any real engagement of entrepreneurs, innovators, and scientists to develop technologies for these communities. Xenophobia creates further reluctance of local engineers and technologists to develop context-appropriate, ethical technologies.

A third reason for a dearth of appropriate technologies designed for the forcibly displaced is a general lack of awareness among innovators about the clinical needs and the socioeconomic environment in which health technologies need to operate.[48] Disaster medicine and humanitarian emergency research has not significantly penetrated areas of technology development. Lack of a nuanced understanding of protracted humanitarian crises,[49] which are different from natural disasters, also limits the scope of technology development and impact. Humanitarian aspects of technology development often don't have a strong focus on chronic ailments[50] and hence remain of limited significance in protracted crises. Curricula in engineering, science, and technology, for example in Pakistan, do not focus on challenges faced by refugees or the stateless within the country, even when these communities are living within an urban community or at a short driving distance from the university campus. The appetite among institutions and students is for new, exciting science, and not for projects that address the pain of a marginalized group.

There is also a sense among scientists and engineers, within both high- and low-income countries, that there are no new questions—worthy of scientific pursuit—unique to forcibly displaced communities.[51]

In their assessment, the issues are only cost and implementation of technology, not new discovery. This assessment discourages new scientists and engineers who are interested in working on the cutting edge, and this assessment is also incorrect. There's a long list of unanswered questions of scientific significance that are unique to the forcibly displaced, for example, the emergence of new diseases[52] due to the built and natural environment in which refugees, migrants, and stateless communities live. Exposure to sewage, urban wastewater, and industrial wastes, in high-density environments lead to development of pathogens less likely to emerge in other settings.[53] The dynamics of disease evolution and spread, which can certainly reach other locations, require basic and applied science investigation and discovery in environments where forcibly displaced communities reside.

There are also important and unanswered questions about the human brain, cognition, mental health, and trauma that are faced by these communities.[54] Studied rigorously, these issues would have long-range implications in improving mental health for many communities around the world. Even in the context of digital health, data privacy questions for the stateless are complex, unique, and have implications for designing ethical systems, which can then be applied to other vulnerable communities.[55]

Increasing the awareness of these issues among potential innovators, engineers, scientists, and technologists faces serious barriers as well. Because of security concerns and potential international embarrassment about their poor treatment of the forcibly displaced (as well as ethical considerations), host countries are often reluctant to allow outside researchers to work and develop a deeper sense of the challenges. The paperwork and bureaucracy required to work in communities that are displaced or marginalized due to state policies[56] makes it difficult for those who somehow overcome the challenges of finances and awareness. Given the nature of the issue, and host governments' policies, working with the stateless is particularly challenging.[57] But financing alone doesn't mean new technologies will be successful or even see their day in the marketplace. Because of siloed approaches[58] when innovators don't engage with social scientists or local communities, and because of limited exposure to ethical analyses, innovators who are able to raise funds lack the ability to fully understand the social context, and hence their technologies are unlikely to be successful in the long-term.

There are also infrastructural challenges that make it difficult for health technologies to survive in the long-term. These range from lack of trained staff to maintain technology, poor access to water and electricity, and unreliable supply chains.[59] In the context of host countries, refugees and the forcibly displaced are at the bottom of the social order, and countries are unlikely to agree on providing them new technologies that aren't available to their citizens.

From time to time, efforts are made by international humanitarian agencies, colleges and universities, and other communities to populate the pipeline of new technologies.[60] There are conferences,[61] meetings, symposia, and hackathons (high-intensity activity by citizens, students, or potential innovators to come up with specific, cost-effective solutions),[62] yet most of them fail to generate new technology for refugees.[63] The general investment, compared to investment needed to see a technology through, is miniscule. Efforts by international aid agencies, including USAID, Gates Foundation, and others, have tried to incentivize groups through programs such as Humanitarian Grand Challenges,[64] but the support provided is relatively small compared to what is needed to bring technology to the marketplace, and scaling of technology remains a serious challenge. Furthermore, programs started by donor agencies supported by governments are always at risk of the changing political winds. Programs started during the Obama administration to incentivize global health technologies were severely curtained in the Trump administration.[65] The lack of continued support—and the disconnect with the local economy—leads to these efforts remaining at a nascent pilot stage. Potential buyers of the technology, agencies such as UNHCR and others, often look for technologies that are already in the marketplace; they are less interested in being part of a new initiative with a promising, but unproven, technology. All these factors ultimately result in health technologies that are largely digital, and the discourse on technologies is limited to information and communication technologies (ICTs). Minimal attention is paid to needed technology infrastructure.

Technology, despite its seemingly endless possibilities, remains out of reach for many.[66] Even for those who can access it, it's an untrustworthy resource. Separated from ethics and equity, it is more likely to be a force for exclusion[67] than a reliable means for accessing quality health care.

Chapter 7
Racism and Discrimination
Impede Access to Health Care

**Rafael sees firsthand Colombia's
discriminatory public health system**

Dr. Vargas looked tired.

Rafael had gotten to know Dr. Vargas through some friends over the last year. In the last few months, Dr. Vargas's confidence in the system had started to shake. He'd always believed in the health system of Colombia, a system that provided quality health care for everyone. In his mind, it was a model for others in the region, and perhaps beyond. Dr. Vargas was committed to the ideals of universal coverage and a state-sponsored safety net. But this idea was no longer working in practice. He felt torn between his values as a physician who chose to stay in the public sector and an increasingly disappearing space for him. When the Venezuelan migrants first started arriving a few years ago, Dr. Vargas felt that this was his opportunity to live by his ideals. He had the tools and the training to support the weak and vulnerable—people he'd always supported and taken an oath to look after, people he believed in when he joined the demonstrations, during medical school, for a better system for all.

The ugly reality, however, had hit hard. The public system in Colombia was built on a model of fee-for-service, or payment-per-event, as the doctors and the hospital administrators called it. That fee-generating event could be a consultation or a surgery, a diagnostic test or a follow-up visit. The state paid for these events. In the last few years, there had been plenty of events in Dr. Vargas's wards, but there had been no payments by the state. The catch in the current model was who came in for the service. If the patient was a Colombian citizen, registered with the national system, the reimbursement model worked fine, and the hospital, doctors, and nurses received a full payment according to a set formula. However, if the patient was a Venezuelan, the system was confusing. In the eyes of the system, all Venezuelans were not equal. Those who had been registered (and had some paperwork) had insurance that would reimburse for some (but not all) services. Exactly what was covered was subjective, depending on the whims, moods, racism, or prior experience of the administrators.

If the patient had no paperwork, the system was unable to pay the doctors. The doctors and nurses could, in principle, treat these patients but could not expect payment. Dr. Vargas—driven by his commitment to equity—had been treating these patients, but was now reaching the end of his goodwill. Despite more than a decade of service in the large hospital in Bogotá, his salary was not guaranteed; it was based on the number of patients he saw and the number of events payable by the state. With a high number of uninsured Venezuelan patients, he was getting paid less and less. While this was frustrating, his own salary was not the only problem; his nurses and support staff were also not getting paid. Dr. Vargas wasn't a wealthy man, but he was still better off than the nurses in his ward, many of whom were less privileged than he was. When a patient was uninsured, no one got paid, not even the technicians who carried out the diagnostic tests.

The hospital administration had recently taken a much harder line when it came to outpatient services and consultations. They had simply started refusing uninsured Venezuelans who arrived for outpatient care. The administrators had less of an option with emergencies: the law said that in case of an emergency, the hospital must care for the patient, regardless of the patient's nationality or ability to pay. However, hospitals had tremendous discretion in how they defined "emergency." Hospital staff—under pressure from the administration—were defining emergencies in a narrower and narrower manner. Hospital administrators were also able to reject potential emergency room visits by requiring formal paperwork or insurance for ambulatory care. Ambulatory care served as the valve into emergency care, and with that valve firmly under the control of administrators, there was little the Venezuelan patients could do. Dr. Vargas was aware of this, but his administrators were unwilling to go any further. They needed their staff to be paid. Their strict stance and unwillingness to accommodate the undocumented Venezuelans had started what the newspapers were now calling *el paseo de la muerte*, the trip of death.[1] The trip of death involved the shuttling of the patient between hospitals, as they were denied care because of their status and lack of appropriate documentation to qualify for insurance, while the patient's condition deteriorated.

Recently, several Venezuelan migrants, suffering not only from chronic conditions but also from COVID-19, were shuttled until they either died on the way to a hospital or at the hospital when it could do little to save them. Sometimes the patients or their families went to court and asked lawyers to get them an emergency relief. The judges were under no pressure to immediately make a decision. Some judges that Rafael worked with, however, were willing to act swiftly and issue orders to save the lives of patients. Both Rafael and Dr. Vargas were aware that, increasingly, it was the courts, and not the hospitals, who were saving the lives of patients.

Dr. Vargas had so far resisted the occasional calls he'd been getting from his friends asking him to start working for a foreign NGO. When a former classmate called last year to offer him a job with an NGO, he dismissed the offer right away. He'd worked in the public system during the darkest days of Colombia. During the civil war he'd been there to treat everyone, even those who wished harm to people like him. He hadn't questioned his decision when others got too scared by narco-terrorism in the streets of Medellín, his hometown. He had worked around the clock to treat wounds and give comfort. He was proud that he didn't leave the country even when he'd had the opportunity and offers of a better salary and a sense of security. He had believed in the public system and had given his life's best years to it. Moving to the NGO sector, to Dr. Vargas, was akin to selling out. He had been unwilling to even consider it.

Dr. Vargas knew that the NGOs were providing primary care and filling a vacuum in the system. More importantly, they provided insurance and payment to the hospitals, which enabled patients to pay for the services, especially during acute emergencies. What the NGOs needed were doctors who wouldn't work in the public system but would work for them instead. In other countries with large numbers of migrants, the international NGOs were often staffed by foreign doctors and nurses. Not in Colombia. The Colombian government made it very difficult for most non-Colombian medical professionals (except those from Venezuela or other neighboring countries) to work in the country.[2] One had to be a Colombian citizen, especially if they wanted to work in urban areas. This meant that even NGOs funded almost exclusively by international donors had to tap into the local pool to staff its clinics.

Dr. Vargas was torn. On one end was his commitment to the public sector and a socially conscious public health system. On the other was the nagging feeling that maybe he was complicit in creating "the trip of death." He'd never thought what he would do if the system he had believed in no longer believed in its own values. Tired and frustrated, Dr. Vargas's wall of resolve to stay in the public system started to crack.

In the most recent call, his friend who'd asked him to consider moving to the NGO last year, made a different argument. He had not even talked about salary and finances. That one was obvious and well-known to all, and was unlikely to work with idealists like Dr. Vargas. The friend had made a moral argument. The NGO doctors, he said, were not discriminating against anyone. They were, to put it bluntly, not racist. Dr. Vargas had not confronted this argument. He had to ask himself what his values were.

Dr. Vargas didn't want to end his career with the feeling that he was, deep down, a racist. In his last meeting with Rafael, he mentioned that he would soon be working for an NGO. There was no excitement in his voice, just resignation and fatigue.

Henry suffers a stroke and must leave the country to access specialty care

Henry never expected to see the health care system from the other side. He was a provider and a caregiver. A healer—spiritual and physical. He had managed to dodge COVID-19. But 2021 would change his perspective permanently.

In April 2021, Henry suffered a stroke. It happened suddenly one afternoon when he was at home in Juba. He could no longer speak, and one side of his body was paralyzed. His daughter rushed him to the public hospital in Juba, but it didn't have the doctors or facilities to treat Henry. So, he was sent back home, where his condition deteriorated quickly.

Henry was unable to eat anything. Several days passed while he continued to wither. To his family he seemed to be slipping away. Juba's public hospitals had nothing available for him. Hospitals in other cities were even less equipped. Those who had the resources, or who worked for a foreign NGO or embassy, would fly out. Henry's family had to do the same to save Henry. The closest option was a hospital in Khartoum, Sudan. There are no roads that can take a patient from Juba to Khartoum, Sudan, about 2,000 kilometers away. The only option was to fly.

Henry didn't have the money for a flight, let alone for a doctor specialized in stroke patients. If Sudan had any form of social safety nets, he was excluded as a noncitizen. His family started to panic and asked around for any help. This was hard, both logistically and emotionally. They had never had to ask for help for themselves. The community was mobilized—friends and family, in country and outside—were asked for help. Extended family members reached out to those whom Henry had taught in the church.

Dr. James, Henry's old friend and supporter, got involved as well. The effort worked, and enough money was raised to fly him to Khartoum to see a doctor at one of the larger facilities. Henry's daughter accompanied him on the trip, and they stayed in Khartoum for about a week. He showed remarkable signs of progress, and his ability to eat gradually returned. In a month's time, he was able to start walking. With some effort, he was able to speak slowly as well. His daughter worked with the hospital in Khartoum to get medicines that would last him at least three months.

Henry now had a newfound appreciation of the challenges his community was facing. He felt for his brother in a way he hadn't felt before. He experienced the complete desert of care around him. Beyond primary care—some of which he was running himself—there was no care. The rich had the capacity to fly out, should there be a need, but the poor had to pray and rely on age-old remedies. Henry also learned that there was little that local doctors could do. They were just as lost in the desert.

Saida's camp has few doctors because of xenophobia

Saida often wondered why there were so few doctors or care providers in Machar Colony. But being a doctor in Machar Colony was not easy. First, you had to be anti-racist. This was a tall ask in a country where Bengalis were viewed with immense suspicion.[3] Fifty years after the break-up of Pakistan, being Bengali meant you were either the target of racist jokes, or viewed as hostile to the ideology of Pakistan. Or both. The poor in the country, regardless of their ethnicity, were often blamed for their ills. Poor and Bengali meant you were the wretched of the earth. As a result, a significant group of people would not be interested in working among Bengalis. In a class- and status-conscious society, working among Bengalis meant family and friends would question one's values, aspirations, and ambition. In the crowded community of Pakistan, where social network and societal approval play a major role in daily life, success is defined in terms of who you hang out with not who needs your help or support. The poor are often accused of being unhygienic and lawless—it is generally assumed they are not educated enough to realize the importance of being law-abiding or they do not care about the sanctity of life. These assumptions act as a deterrent to young women to work in the colony. A dirty place, with poor people, was no place for girls from good families.

Newly minted doctors, in Karachi or elsewhere, preferred jobs that either offered attractive salaries or provided training opportunities in innovative hospitals with new equipment. The most successful were those who studied abroad—preferably in the United States. A series of carefully curated steps were needed to land a residency, and a successful career, in Europe or the United States.[4] Many medical students who studied on subsidized education left the country right after graduation. Others, who willingly or unwillingly stayed within the system, often chose training in places where they could be mentored by clinicians recognized for their acumen, intelligence, renown, and connections. Machar Colony offered none of this. Helping Saida or her brother provided no incentive for most clinicians in the country.

Working in Machar Colony was the exact opposite of the right career move. In addition to the community of people who were looked down upon, there were no large hospitals, no mentors, and no colleagues immersed in research. There were no seminars, no visiting foreign doctors, no grand rounds. Most importantly, there were no public hospitals to work at, which meant that their years working in Machar

Colony would not count towards their service in the public sector. Because of poor literacy, and lack of opportunities for even basic education, the Bengali community was unable to produce its own doctors. They relied completely on outside agencies to set up the clinics and provide doctors and medical staff.

All of this meant that there weren't many doctors in Machar Colony. Each clinic usually had only one doctor, if they had any at all. The doctors were either between jobs (and wanted to maintain their connection to medicine while earning a decent living) or were supplementing their income by working in multiple clinics. The NGOs in Machar Colony paid reasonably well. While the salaries certainly weren't at the level of private practice salaries, they were still comparable to what other nonprofit clinics in the city were paying. The only issue was that the doctors had to deal with people they didn't like very much.

Doctors were able to work in multiple clinics because the clinics were typically open only until two o'clock in the afternoon (or in one case, until five o'clock) and only on weekdays. No emergency calls and no requirements to work in the evenings, nights, or weekends meant that the doctors could work at other clinics outside the colony. The cases they had to deal with were also not particularly hard. There were no surgeries in the colony clinics and no ICUs. There was, therefore, no need for a highly sanitized environment, or dependence on sophisticated equipment that required training or maintenance. There was no need to stay up-to-date with the latest research and practices. Yet, despite the relatively easy workload and a decent salary, few ventured. And those who did join didn't stay long. Often they left after a few months, once they found a better job. Some left while making caustic remarks about Bengalis being responsible for their ill fortune and being the source of all their own problems.

Every now and then, there were exceptions.

Dr. Samina has worked in Machar Colony since 2017 and, despite the immense challenge of poverty in the community and racism, she wasn't ready to give up. Dr. Samina herself had not grown up in the colony. In fact she didn't even grow up in Karachi. She was from Hyderabad, the second largest city in the province, about 160 kilometers northeast of the colony. After she finished her residency, she was told by a friend about the opening in the colony's clinic. She applied, spoke to the local organization running the clinic, and felt that this was her calling. She wasn't ethnically Bengali and didn't have any interaction with Bengalis while growing up. Guided by her spirituality and her faith, she felt it was her responsibility to serve those who were needy and without substantial resources. For a few hours each day, she worked at the free clinic in the colony. At other times, she treated patients in a working-class neighborhood of Manzoor Colony.

After working in Machar Colony for four years, Dr. Samina started to feel part of the community. She worked as a primary care doctor seeing only women and children. But given the dearth of clinicians and professionals who chose to interact with the community, she was more than a doctor diagnosing or prescribing treatments. She routinely dispensed advice about matters beyond the realm of health, ranging from schooling to urban environments, from marital conflicts to troubles with in-laws.

Dr. Samina's patients represented the state's failure and the degrading environmental conditions in which people were forced to live.[5] Her clinic was located in a dense neighborhood, where people lived with no sanitation, limited nutrition, and occupational hazards in the unregulated fishing industry. Skin diseases[6] were common all year round. Saida and her whole family had battled such infections for as long as she could remember. This was, in part, due to the poorly run fisheries, where nearly everyone worked.[7] Rashes, skin lesions, and infections were further exacerbated by sanitation issues in the colony. Respiratory infections were also common, driven in part by dust and air pollution and in part by seasonal infections and allergies. Pregnancy complications due to poor diet, stress, and limited access to prenatal visits were routine. During the summer and fall, dengue fever, driven in part by mosquitoes breeding in stagnant water, affected her patients, and some got really sick. In the rainy season it was a different set of ailments: stomach bugs and gastrointestinal problems. Hepatitis C continues to be a grave concern.[8] Given the dearth of options for the women, she saw as many as sixty patients during her four-hour workday. She had to know her own limits as a community doctor, but more importantly she had to know her patients' limits in their ability to access the facilities.

Dr. Samina was frustrated and angry by the crippling poverty, lack of education, racism, and exclusion. She often wondered how things could change when people had nothing to eat. But she was more troubled by her own professional community—the doctors she had trained with, the clinicians she knew socially. The sense of entitlement among her peers bothered her tremendously. At times she felt lonely, not sure whether her work would lead to any permanent change. Xenophobia had erased Saida and her folks from the worldview of the state and its most accomplished professionals. Dr. Samina knew that the state had failed but unfortunately so had her peers, who—while speaking endlessly in conferences all across the world about the grand ideals of medicine—were failing to see their own racism.

Racism and discrimination are permanent barriers to accessing health care

In his diary for September 7, 1967, Pakistan's military dictator and president, Field Marshal Muhammad Ayub Khan wrote dismissively about the Bengali population of East Pakistan: "how to save people who do not want to be saved"; "God has been very unkind to us in giving the sort of neighbors and compatriots we have. We could not think of a worst combination. Hindus and Bengalis."[9] Finally, he made his intentions clear about how to treat them should they continue to complain about the injustice from the Western part of the country (where Ayub Khan was located) and protest. "Rivers of blood will flow if need be, unhappily."[10]

President Ayub Khan is no ordinary figure in Pakistan's history. He is viewed by some, including many dictators who followed him and political leaders with pro-military sympathies, as the model leader.[11] He is credited with overseeing the glorious period of Pakistan, the so-called Decade of Development, from 1958 to 1969.[12]

While he is long gone, and had a rather unceremonious and disgraceful exit from office, his sentiments about Bengalis still echo loudly in the country. In a recent short television documentary about the condition of the stateless Bengalis in Pakistan, the sentiment was clear.[13] When several citizens of Karachi were asked whether there should be a CNIC card, or citizenship, for the Bengalis who live in Pakistan, the answer was an emphatic *no*. That sentiment remains strong not just in Karachi but all over Pakistan. The argument goes that Bengalis have their "own" country—never mind that as many as 80 percent of the community members of Machar Colony were born in Pakistan, consider themselves Pakistani, and have never visited Bangladesh, or that Bangladesh has shown no interest in taking in hundreds of thousands of ethnic Bengalis based in Pakistan. The country of Bangladesh (like any other country) has little interest in bringing in people who are poor, illiterate, and unskilled.[14]

The environment of hostility and xenophobia is not just on the fringes of debates. It consumes all sectors of society. Many doctors and nurses, public health professionals, and health bureaucrats view the stateless and the forcibly displaced as outsiders and usurpers of benefits. While this sentiment is particularly targeted at refugees and the stateless, IDPs are not immune from it either. The military operations of the early 2000s in the northwestern regions of Pakistan created millions of IDPs living in camps or in cities, and there were severe restrictions on their movement, which was driven by a sense of suspicion and racism.[15]

When IDPs are located in an area of a different tribe or culture, xenophobia is palpable; but even when they are not, class consciousness influences how their access to health care is viewed. Because they are poor, others assume they are likely to have no sense of hygiene or awareness about good health practices. Often, the sentiment expressed by President Ayub Khan (that no one can save people who do not want to be saved) is echoed by others, who suggest that the lack of initiative among the poor, combined with their own corruption, is the cause of their misery. People in Pakistan aren't the only ones who commit the racist act of accusing the poor of self-inflicted misery; American politicians, too, routinely blame Black poverty on Black culture.[16]

This sense that the poor are responsible for their misfortune drives the view of many medical professionals in host countries. There is a sense among the local population (more than among foreign aid workers, although they aren't immune from racism) that the poor health of the refugees is due to their own actions. While poverty, exclusion, and lack of access to good services do have strong, negative influences on health outcomes, this is not universally true. For example, recent work in Lahore, Pakistan's second largest city, showed that antimicrobial resistance patterns among Afghan refugees were similar, or better, than resistance patterns among local residents.[17]

Lack of cultural awareness, and poor representation of the local community (e.g., few South Sudanese doctors work in refugee camps in Uganda, and almost none are ethnically Bengali in Machar Colony) further reinforces cultural stereotypes. In places where local doctors are able to speak the language, or are from the community (e.g., Native American doctors working within the US Indian Health Service), outcomes can improve through a system of understanding, trust, and relationship building.[18] In the absence of local integration, privileged medical professionals often use a patronizing attitude, combined with a sense of pity, and they don't discuss actual problem-solving using a holistic approach to health. Tackling this general sense of cultural disconnect, however, is no easy task because of a lack of resources, programs, and efforts to build technical capacity among the forcibly displaced. Racism, along with suspicion,[19] continues to undermine such efforts, and most efforts are made at an informal, nongovernmental level rather than one that has the full support of the state.

Under normal circumstances, doctors and nurses often do not choose to work with the forcibly displaced or the stateless. There are strong disincentives to do so. However, under extreme circumstances, they may not have many options. When the entire health care system collapses (due to conflict and active targeting of health services), doctors are forced to work for international NGOs or humanitarian agencies as their only option to generate income. For example, as a result of the conflict in Yemen, the entire public sector has nearly collapsed. Doctors are among many groups in the public sector who have not been paid in years. While some continued coming to work at the hospitals, others eventually gave up on the system. There was a demand in the international humanitarian sector, serving as primary care doctors in mobile health units. Some doctors, who previously worked as specialists or surgeons, accepted these jobs. The doctors I spoke to in Yemen felt a sense of loss, and were unenthusiastic about working in these mobile units. Their lack of motivation was evident to their patients, who depended on the mobile health units; these patients felt that the doctors in these units were not really interested in hearing, or solving, their problems.

Local doctors and medical professionals who find the moral courage to work among the dispossessed by choice and desire, despite social pressures not to, are also at risk of burning out due to systemic barriers and high stress.[20] There is no real local institutional support for these doctors. They are often the only doctor in a particular unit, and they have to work and survive within academic, professional, and intellectual islands. There are no professional organizations, communities, or groups that can provide mentorship, guidance, or support to handle complex challenges. These health care professionals find themselves tackling problems well beyond what they are trained for. They are not just acting as medical doctors but also as therapists, counselors and social workers. In addition, they have to address issues of logistics, supplies, and maintenance of equipment. Since there is no real support from the system, the pressure has an impact on their practice, and the time they devote to their patients. Some doctors are able to handle this; others burn out and move on to something easier. Local NGOs, and refugee-led organizations that can provide quality care with a deeper understanding of the social and cultural context,[21] are also often at risk of losing their funding, which acts as a deterrent against recruiting or retaining outside health professionals.

The jobs with international NGOs are competitive and coveted, and local doctors who are able to work for international agencies do better, both financially and in terms of peer support. However, international organizations are not always able to work in local communities and are at the whim of the government to start and continue their operations.[22] Depending on the political winds, they are often the first target of an authoritarian regime that views them as foreign agents of unfriendly governments.

While salaries, benefits, and consistent, stable employment matter to medical professionals who care for the most vulnerable, the factors that result in a dysfunctional system that continues to fail the patients is the lack of an empathetic institutional structure, combined with inherent racism in the system.

Conclusion

Rafael, Henry, and Saida are all journeying on their paths, although none believe that they are settled.

Rafael is still in Bogotá, working with a few different NGOs and trying to help Venezuelan migrants navigate the system. It has been five years since he left Venezuela. He doesn't see going back as a viable option anytime soon. He misses his home terribly, but he believes Venezuela has gone too far down the road of collapse and that it will take a long time, perhaps longer than his lifetime, for it to return to some kind of normalcy. His immediate hope, and his greatest desire, is a reunion with his daughters in Bogotá. However, with new curbs on movement since the beginning of the pandemic, and with limited options for Venezuelans to come to Colombia, that seems unlikely in the near future.

Henry's brother, Solomon lived with him in Juba, and showed early signs of improvement. For the first few months, he spoke a bit more and ate better, which made Henry happy. Henry had created a system of well-wishers and prayer groups that provided his brother with counseling and moral support. The network also helped get medicines for

Solomon when needed; the medicines were available in Juba, although they're not free. This network had been critical for caring for Solomon, especially because Henry had to deal with his own health issues. In March 2022, however, Solomon's health took a turn for the worse, and he started deteriorating rapidly. He died on March 19, 2022, leaving Henry to take care of not just the funeral arrangements but also his brother's family.

Henry's own health has gotten much better in the last few months. He is able to talk without any discomfort and can walk without a stick. He is communicating with friends abroad on WhatsApp. This recovery for Henry, unfortunately, has been neither easy nor cheap. He still needs follow-up visits, which can only happen in Sudan, and he is dependent on friends and family, particularly those who live in the United States and Europe, to send him money. During the pandemic, medical expense fees have gone up and so have flight costs. A follow-up visit to Khartoum can cost as much as six thousand dollars (US), including flights and private clinics. Yet, Henry feels that he has a greater calling now to work for his family and his people and provide them with both medical care and spiritual guidance. He has started, once again, to travel to smaller towns for his missionary work, and is eager to expand his engagement with the church.

Saida's brother, Tanvir, is doing much better. To the staff at the clinic, he seems like a completely different person. He talks freely, smiles when he talks, and doesn't look down when spoken to. His personal appearance has changed for the better as well. In the fall of 2021, the clinic staff told him that he was now well enough that he did not need any more appointments, although he was always welcome anytime. He no longer goes to the mental health clinic, but he still goes to the legal aid clinic. His CNIC issue is still unresolved, although he has found a job through some contacts, and seems happier than ever before. Saida, while more relaxed than she has been in a while, knows that Tanvir is perhaps only one bad experience away from falling deeper into despair. She is tired and anxious but more energetic and determined to get her brother and son the CNIC they deserve. Seeing a transformation in Tanvir, she is more hopeful about the future.

| Over the course of my research for this book and talking to people in camps, urban informal settlements, slums, and temporary dwellings in dozens of countries, the most striking thing was how focusing solely on one particular aspect of the challenge, while ignoring others, was making the problem much worse. It became clear to me that the barriers to health care access among the forcibly displaced and the stateless cannot be viewed in isolation. This means that a campaign focusing on a single disease (e.g., an infection) may help some people but is unlikely to change the overall state of health care access. In the long run it is going to make matters worse for everyone. Childhood vaccinations are critically important, but children also need nutrition, schooling, and a hygienic environment. Their parents and caregivers also need to be protected against diseases, and taken care of when they are ill.

The current system of funding health care for the stateless often looks at individual challenges and prioritizes vertical programs. That is convenient for fundraising and self-reporting against a series of impact metrics, and international agencies are increasingly built around this approach, but health care cannot be partitioned into neat boxes of diseases. Those who have underlying conditions, like diabetes and cardiovascular ailments, which have nothing to do with a virus, are far more likely to have poor outcomes when colonized by a viral infection like COVID-19. Those who are malnourished in camps do worse than those who have better nutrition when both groups are faced with a bacterial infection. The partition between communicable and noncommunicable diseases is both arbitrary and dangerous, and one that is unlikely to bring a permanent positive change. Those of us who are fortunate and privileged do not see ourselves as living in this binary world of infection or noncommunicable diseases, so why should we view others in this way? Access to health care therefore needs to be integrated across ailments and conditions, integrated with education and the right to work, and viewed first and foremost as a human right.

Just as access to health care cannot be viewed from the isolated, and myopic, lens of a single ailment, neither should the access be looked at from a purely economic lens. Access should not be predicated on the fact that if we provide access to quality health care, we are likely to have a strong workforce. Arguments to support refugees are often made in economic and labor terms, and it is said that refugees are good for the economy because they are entrepreneurial, or because they work hard.[1] While that itself may be true, this policy rationale is inherently exclusionary. This line of argument would deprioritize anyone who is not part of the labor market, such as persons with a serious health condition, the elderly, or those with any disability. This argument also means in countries where there is no shortage of labor (for example, the stateless Bengalis in Pakistan), there is little incentive to help the stateless since they will not add any real economic value.

Ultimately, access to health care among the marginalized, vulnerable, and disenfranchised has to be connected to human and civil rights. Disconnecting it from basic rights to education, employment, and safety is not helpful. Health care cannot be chopped up into neat squares of diseases, or mandates that focus only on a particular age group or a single nutritional deficiency. The approach, first and foremost, has to be rooted in anti-racism. This reframing of the problem would require rethinking how we think of other people who may not look like us, and whose mere presence around us makes us uncomfortable. This is a big ask, particularly in a climate of xenophobia, anxiety, and nativism. Yet, two recent developments have opened up the possibility for change.

The first is the global conversation on anti-racism catalyzed by events in the United States and beyond in light of the murder of George Floyd in May 2020. The recent movement and associated discussions are asking tough (but correct) questions to challenge our existing notions of equity and inclusion.

The second is the global COVID-19 pandemic, which laid bare the cracks that were already there in the society and how health care was made available and accessed. We were either not ready to see these fissures of inequity in health care availability and access, or we weren't interested in seeing them. In cities and towns all across the world, socioeconomic disparities have shown that those who were already disadvantaged did worse than those who were privileged. The privileged had more immediate access to health care, better access to information, and the ability to prioritize health without the risk of losing a job. The pandemic has also provided us with clear evidence about the necessity of systems thinking, and understanding that access to health care requires a deeper analysis of equity and a foundation of empathy. It has also underscored the need to think beyond discoveries, technologies, and institutions, and has laid bare our own limitations in understanding human behavior, trust, and how we view information.

I hope that out of the pandemic and the movement for equity and justice, we will be able to see not just ourselves in the mirror and commit to change, but have the mirror be clean enough to see those around us who have remained invisible for so long.

Acknowledgments

I started working on this book nearly six years ago. It was conversations in the camps, informal settlements, clinics, and classrooms that framed the ideas that underpin this book. But halfway through my research and writing, a virus and our hubris changed the world. The conversations that were previously taking place in person, in coffee shops, labs, clinics, and homes had to move to the virtual world of WhatsApp and Zoom. Despite tremendous anxiety and near-permanent uncertainty, the main characters in this book and their families were always available to speak to me. I do not have, or will ever have, the words to thank them for their generosity and their belief in this project.

I am also grateful to my friends, colleagues, and research partners from all over the world. This book is a result of their constant support. They were patient with my repeated questions, available to talk at all times of the day and night, and ready to correct my assumptions. In Pakistan, Tahera Hasan and the team at Imkaan (in particular, Dr. Samina Kanwar and Ayesha Sami) were instrumental to my work and my understanding of the complex challenges facing the stateless. In Colombia,

Dr. Oscar Acevedo, Dr. German Casas, and their colleagues opened many doors for me. In South Sudan, Dr. Wani Mena connected me with Henry and was my mentor every step of the way. In Zimbabwe, Dr. Saranna Ammeer was generous with her time and has always been just a phone call away, whether she is in town or halfway across the world. Dr. Najwa Dheeb in Yemen remains a true inspiration with her energy, her work ethic, and her unwavering commitment to human dignity.

This work would not have been possible without the wisdom, expertise, and experience of historians, urban planners, clinicians, anthropologists, and public policy experts who were my guides in various parts of my research. Lara Alshawawreh, Jeff Crisp, Jessica Goudeau, Baher Ibrahim, Anne Irfan, Ulrike Krause, Elisa Mason, Lara Mourad, Kelsey Norman, Laura Robson, and Benjamin Thomas White shared their knowledge and experience generously and were always available to guide me.

Closer to home, my colleagues and students at Boston University were always eager to help and were there for me every step of the way. I cannot ask for better colleagues than Carrie Preston and Marina Lazetic. They helped me in countless ways as I grappled with questions, needed to sharpen my arguments, or challenge my own biases. I am indebted to both of them for so much. They make me a better person every day.

My students Maria Santarelli and Alexandra Van Waes helped me with research in Colombia during some of the darkest days of the pandemic. Nisrine Rahmaoui, Rana Hussein, and Carly Ching read the manuscript and gave invaluable advice. As always, my research group was there for me as I navigated travel, teaching, research, and writing. Financial support from the Guggenheim Foundation made this research possible. I am also deeply grateful to the Schooner Foundation for their support. They believed in me and were among the first to provide essential resources as I started this work.

I was fortunate to work with an all-star team at Johns Hopkins University Press. Robin Coleman is the kind of editor we all dream of. He is encouraging, patient, and kind and always has something very meaningful to add. Susan Matheson worked her magic on the copy-editing front; the final product is much better thanks to her advice and editing. Charles Dibble's support during the final stages of production was essential.

Family has always been the most important part of all my projects. My brother Qasim, my sisters Rabia and Fakiha, and their families have always been there for me. Their love is a permanent source of joy in my life. I am also incredibly fortunate to receive immense love and support from my in-laws. I am grateful for all that they do for me.

A lot changed in my life and my work during the pandemic, but one thing never changed—even for an instant. It was the constant love and support of my family. They are the light of my life. Our son, Rahem, and our daughter, Samah, are the reason our home is bright, cheerful, and always my favorite place to be.

Afreen is not just the love of my life, my soulmate, and my life partner but also the first person with whom I talk about all of my research ideas. Her love and support are the foundation on which I stand. None of my work would be possible without her.

Notes

Introduction

1. For more on the Hathora group and conspiracies it fueled, see Jafar Rizvi and Riaz Sohail, "Hathora (Hammer) Group: What Was the Group that Spread Fear and Terror on the Streets of Karachi and Where Did It Go?," *BBC Urdu*, April 5, 2022, https://www.bbc.com/urdu/pakistan -60062067.

Chapter 1
Current Situations of Forcibly Displaced Persons

1. Ewald Scharfenberg, "Maduro Sugiere Que los que Reciben las Viviendas del Estado Paguen por Ellas" ["Maduro Suggests That Those Who Receive State Housing Pay for It"], *El Pais*, May 16, 2013, https://elpais .com/internacional/2013/05/17/actualidad/1368753065_850617.html.

2. "Disorder on the Border: Keeping the Peace between Colombia and Venezuela," International Crisis Group (website), December 14, 2020, https://www.crisisgroup.org/latin-america-caribbean/andes/colombia /84-disorder-border-keeping-peace-between-colombia-and-venezuela.

3. M. A. Barusya, "Uganda's Refugee Policy: A Case of Bidi Bidi Camp" (PhD diss., Makerere University, 2018).

4. A. Arnold and M. LeRiche, *South Sudan: From Revolution to Independence* (Oxford University Press, 2013).

5. E. Thomas, *South Sudan: A Slow Liberation* (Bloomsbury Publishing, 2015).

6. Ashley Quarcoo, "A Brief Guide to South Sudan's Fragile Peace," Carnegie Endowment for International Peace, December 12, 2019, https://carnegieendowment.org/2019/12/12/brief-guide-to-south-sudan -s-fragile-peace-pub-80570.

7. Alex Adaku, James Okello, Blakeley Lowry, Jeremy C. Kane, Stephen Alderman, Seggane Musisi, and Wietse A. Tol, "Mental Health and Psychosocial Support for South Sudanese Refugees in Northern Uganda: A Needs and Resource Assessment," *Conflict and Health* 10, no. 1 (2016): 1–10.

8. Aziz Atamanov, Theresa Beltramo, Peter Waita, and Nobuo Yoshida, "COVID-19 Socioeconomic Impact Worsens for Refugees in Uganda," World Bank, July 14, 2021, https://blogs.worldbank.org/dev4peace /covid-19-socioeconomic-impact-worsens-refugees-uganda.

9. "COVID-19 poses a major threat to the life and welfare of refugees in Uganda," Relief Web, June 17, 2021, https://reliefweb.int/report/uganda /covid-19-poses-major-threat-life-and-welfare-refugees-uganda.

10. This issue has been documented elsewhere as well; see for example: Paul Bukuluki, Peter Kisaakye, Symon Peter Wandiembe, and Samuel Besigwa, "Suicide Ideation and Psychosocial Distress among Refugee Adolescents in Bidibidi Settlement in West Nile, Uganda," *Discover Psychology* 1, no. 1 (2021): 1–9.

11. Hajira Maryam, "Stateless and Helpless: The Plight of Ethnic Bengalis in Pakistan," *Al Jazeera*, September 29, 2021, https://www.aljazeera.com /amp/features/2021/9/29/stateless-ethnic-bengalis-pakistan.

12. Mansoor Raza, "Documentation and Analysis of the Current Housing Trends in Machar Colony in Karachi, Pakistan," *Journal of Research in Architecture and Planning* 26, no. 2 (2019): 19–33, https://jrap.neduet.edu .pk/arch-journal/JRAP_2019(SecondIssue)/03.pdf.

13. Even the president of Pakistan at the time believed this. See for example, Mohammad Ayub Khan, *Diaries of Field Marshal Mohammad Ayub Khan, 1966–1972* (Oxford University Press, 2007), 144–46.

14. Muhammad Hamid Zaman, Tahera Hasan, and Janki Bhatt, "Invisible People, Visible Barriers: Healthcare Access for and among Ethnic Bengalis in Pakistan," *Statelessness & Citizenship Review* 4, no. 2 (2022):

286–92, https://statelessnessandcitizenshipreview.com/index.php /journal/article/view/357.

15. Rakib Al Hasan, "Bengalis in Pakistan: A Neglected Community Crying for Recognition," *South Asia Monitor*, June 18, 2021, https://www .southasiamonitor.org/spotlight/bengalis-pakistan-neglected-community -crying-recognition.

16. "Special Report on Informal Housing," *The New Humanitarian*, November 10, 2003, https://www.thenewhumanitarian.org/fr/node/190448.

17. Raza, "Documentation and Analysis of the Current Housing Trends."

18. Arif Hasan, "Why Karachi Floods," *Dawn*, September 6, 2020, https:// www.dawn.com/news/1578061.

19. Xari Jalil, "50 Years of Statelessness: The Bengalis of Macchar [*sic*] Colony," Voicepk.net, December 27, 2021, https://voicepk.net/2021/12 /50-years-of-statelessness-the-bengalis-of-macchar-colony/.

20. Rauf Ansari, "Easy Access Fuels Ever-stronger Drug Addiction in Youth," *Daily Times*, May 5, 2019, https://dailytimes.com.pk/388347/easy-access -fuels-ever-stronger-drug-addiction-in-youth/.

21. "Refugee Statistics," UNHCR, https://www.unrefugees.org/refugee-facts /statistics/.

22. "Forced Displacement Passes 80 Million by Mid-2020 as COVID-19 Tests Refugee Protection Globally," UNHCR, December 9, 2020, https://www .unhcr.org/en-us/news/press/2020/12/5fcf94a04/forced-displacement -passes-80-million-mid-2020-covid-19-tests-refugee-protection.html.

23. Sonja Fransen and Hein De Haas, "Trends and Patterns of Global Refugee Migration," *Population and Development Review* 48, no. 1 (2022): 97–128.

24. E. O. Abuya, U. Krause, and L. Mayblin, "The Neglected Colonial Legacy of the 1951 Refugee Convention, *International Migration* 59, no. 4 (2021): 265–67.

25. Gil Loescher, *The UNHCR and World Politics* (Oxford University Press, 2001), 43–46.

26. Pia Oberoi, "South Asia and the Creation of the International Refugee Regime," *Refuge* 19 (2000): 36.

27. Loescher, UNHCR and World Politics, 105–34.

28. Benjamin Thomas White, "Talk of an 'Unprecedented' Number of Refugees Is Wrong—and Dangerous," *The New Humanitarian*, October 3, 2019, https://www.thenewhumanitarian.org/opinion/2019/10/03 /unprecedented-number-refugees-wrong-dangerous.

29. William Henderson, "The Refugees in India and Pakistan" *Journal of International Affairs* (1953): 57–65.
30. Refugee Data Finder, UNHCR, https://www.unhcr.org/refugee -statistics/insights/explainers/forcibly-displaced-pocs.html.
31. "Internally Displaced Persons: The Role of the UNHCR," UNHCR Standing Committee, June 20, 2000, https://www.unhcr.org/3ae68d150.pdf.
32. Natalia Baal and Laura Ronkainen, "Obtaining Representative Data on IDPs: Challenges and Recommendations," UNHCR, April 30, 2017.
33. Mary Mostafanezhad, "'Getting in Touch with Your Inner Angelina': Celebrity Humanitarianism and the Cultural Politics of Gendered Generosity in Volunteer Tourism," *Third World Quarterly* 34, no. 3 (2013): 485–99.
34. See for example: Azmat Khan, "Ghost Students, Ghost Teachers, Ghost Schools," *BuzzFeed News*, July 8, 2015, https://www.buzzfeednews.com /article/azmatkhan/the-big-lie-that-helped-justify-americas-war-in -afghanistan; and Anand Gopal, *No Good Men among the Living: America, the Taliban, and the War through Afghan Eyes* (Metropolitan books, 2014).
35. Roger Zetter, "Introduction: Unlocking the Protracted Displacement of Refugees and Internally Displaced Persons: An Overview," *Refugee Survey Quarterly* 30, no. 4 (2011): 1–13.
36. Patricia Hynes, *Introducing Forced Migration* (Routledge, 2021).
37. "Country Profile: Colombia," Internal Displacement Monitoring Centre, May 18, 2022, https://www.internal-displacement.org/countries/colombia.
38. Juan Esteban Zea, "Internal Displacement in Colombia: Violence, Resettlement, and Resistance" (master's thesis, Portland State University, 2010).
39. Roland Popp, "War in Yemen: Revolution and Saudi Intervention," *CSS Analyses in Security Policy* 175 (2015).
40. Noor Elahi, "Militancy Conflicts and Displacement in Swat Valley of Pakistan: Analysis of Transformation of Social and Cultural Network," *International Journal of Humanities and Social Science* 5, no. 3 (2015): 226–36; and Najam U. Din, *Internal Displacement in Pakistan: Contemporary Challenges*, Human Rights Commission of Pakistan, 2010, https://dev.humanitarianlibrary.org/sites/default/files/2014/02/22.pdf.
41. Thomas McGee, "Recognising Stateless Refugees," *Forced Migration Review* 65 (November 2020): 45–47.

42. Antara Datta, "The Repatriation of 1973 and the Re-making of Modern South Asia," *Contemporary South Asia* 19, no. 1 (2011): 61–74.

43. Judy Austin, Samantha Guy, Louise Lee-Jones, Therese McGinn, and Jennifer Schlecht, "Reproductive Health: A Right for Refugees and Internally Displaced Persons," *Reproductive Health Matters* 16, no. 31 (2008): 10–21.

44. Walter Kälin and Hannah Entwisle Chapuisat, "Guiding Principle 28: The Unfulfilled Promise to End Protracted Internal Displacement," *International Journal of Refugee Law* 30, no. 2 (2018): 243–68.

45. C. M. Bailliet, "Protection of Refugees, Returnees, Migrants, and Internally Displaced Persons against Racism, Xenophobia, and Discriminatory Practices," July 5, 2018, https://ssrn.com/abstract=3481195.

46. Peter Heudtlass, Niko Speybroeck, and Debarati Guha-Sapir, "Excess Mortality in Refugees, Internally Displaced Persons and Resident Populations in Complex Humanitarian Emergencies (1998–2012): Insights from Operational Data," *Conflict and Health* 10, no. 1 (2016): 1–11.

47. Peter Gatrell, *The Making of the Modern Refugee* (Oxford University Press, 2013), 21–52.

48. Laura Robson, "What Are Refugee Camps For?," *Current Affairs*, January 7, 2020, https://www.currentaffairs.org/2020/01/what-are-refugee-camps-for.

49. Rebecca Napier-Moore, "Entrenched Relations and the Permanence of Long-term Refugee Camp Situations," working paper no. 28, Sussex Centre for Migration, 2005.

50. Romola Sanyal, "Refugees and the City: An Urban Discussion," *Geography Compass* 6, no. 11 (2012): 633–44.

51. Denielle Amparado, Helen Dempster, and Imran Khan Laghari, "With US Withdrawal, Rights of Afghan Refugees Hang in the Balance," Center for Global Development, Report on Afghan Refugees in Pakistan, August 25, 2021, https://www.cgdev.org/blog/us-withdrawal-rights-afghan-refugees-pakistan-hang-balance.

52. Muhammad Abbas Khan, "Pakistan's Urban Refugees: Steps towards Self-reliance," *Forced Migration Review* 63 (February 2020), 50–52.

53. "Myth and Facts: Where Do Refugees Live?," UNHCR (website), August 9, 2018, https://www.unrefugees.org/news/myths-facts-where-do-refugees-live/.

54. Karen Jacobsen, "Refugees and Asylum Seekers in Urban Areas: A Livelihoods Perspective," *Journal of Refugee Studies* 19, no. 3 (2006): 273–86.

55. Chinedu Temple Obi, "How Refugees' Decision to Live In or Outside a Camp Affects their Quality of Life," World Bank (blog), March 2, 2021, https://blogs.worldbank.org/dev4peace/how-refugees-decision-live-or-outside-camp-affects-their-quality-life.

56. Romola Sanyal, "From Camps to Urban Refugees: Reflections on Research Agendas," *International Journal of Urban and Regional Research* (2016), https://www.ijurr.org/spotlight-on/the-urban-refugee-crisis-reflections-on-cities-citizenship-and-the-displaced/from-camps-to-urban-refugees-reflections-on-research-agendas/.

57. Mohamad Alloush, J. Edward Taylor, Anubhab Gupta, Ruben Irvin Rojas Valdes, and Ernesto Gonzalez-Estrada, "Economic Life in Refugee Camps," *World Development* 95 (2017): 334–47.

58. "Yemen: The Implications of Forced Immobility," Policy Paper, Internal Displacement Monitoring Centre, June 2020, https://www.internal-displacement.org/sites/default/files/publications/documents/202006-yemen-policy-paper.pdf.

59. Irit Katz, Diana Martín, and Claudio Minca, eds., *Camps Revisited: Multifaceted Spatialities of a Modern Political Technology* (Rowman & Littlefield, 2018).

60. Tom Scott-Smith and Mark E. Breeze, eds., *Structures of Protection? Rethinking Refugee Shelter*, Forced Migration, vol. 39 (Berghahn Books, 2020).

61. Miriam Orcutt, Clare Shortall, Sarah Walpole, Aula Abbara, Sylvia Garry, Rita Issa, Alimuddin Zumla, and Ibrahim Abubakar, eds., *Handbook of Refugee Health: For Healthcare Professionals and Humanitarians Providing Care to Forced Migrants* (CRC Press, 2021).

62. Hind Sharif, "Refugee-led Humanitarianism in Lebanon's Shatila Camp," *Forced Migration Review* 57 (2018): 10–12.

63. UNHCR Data Report on Refugees in Uganda, UNHCR (website), Uganda Comprehensive Refugee Response Portal, https://data.unhcr.org/en/country/uga.

64. Felipe Gómez Isa, "The Forced Displacement of Indigenous Peoples in Colombia," *Global Campus Human Rights Journal* 2, no. 1 (2018): 77–95.

65. Amar Guriro, "A Portrait of a Karachi Slum during a Heatwave," The Third Pole (website), May 28, 2018, https://www.thethirdpole.net/en/livelihoods/a-portrait-of-a-karachi-slum-during-a-heatwave/.

66. Kelsey P. Norman, *Reluctant Reception: Refugees, Migration and Governance in the Middle East and North Africa* (Cambridge University Press, 2020), 147–68.

67. Maria Vincenza Desiderio, "Integrating Refugees into Host Country Labor Markets: Challenges and Policy Options," Migration Policy Institute, 2016.

68. Gerasimos Tsourapas, "The Syrian Refugee Crisis and Foreign Policy Decision-making in Jordan, Lebanon, and Turkey," *Journal of Global Security Studies* 4, no. 4 (2019): 464–48.

69. Juline Beaujouan and Amjed Rasheed, "An Overview of the Syrian Refugee Crisis in Lebanon and Its Socio-economic Impact," in *Syrian Crisis, Syrian Refugees: Voices from Jordan and Lebanon*, ed. Juline Beaujouan and Amjed Rasheed, Mobility & Politics series (Palgrave Pivot Cham, 2020), 35–46.

70. Diego Chaves-González and Carlos Echevarría Estrada, "Venezuelan Migrants and Refugees in Latin America and the Caribbean: A Regional Profile," Migration Policy Institute, 2020.

71. Benjamin J. Roth, "Exploring the Local Organizational Response to Venezuelan Migrants in Colombia," Justice Sector Training, Research and Coordination (JUSTRAC) Research Report, 2019, 1–49.

72. Norman, *Reluctant Reception*.

73. Veronika Fajth, Özge Bilgili, Craig Loschmann, and Melissa Siegel, "How Do Refugees Affect Social Life in Host Communities? The Case of Congolese Refugees in Rwanda," *Comparative Migration Studies* 7, no. 1 (2019): 1–21.

74. Maheshvari Naidu and Abigail Benhura, "Internal Displacement and Forced Migration within Zimbabwe: An Overview," *Journal of Social Development in Africa* 30, no. 1 (2015): 147–69.

75. Anthony Pahnke, "The World's Definition of 'Refugee' Shortchanges Economic Migrants," *LA Times*, January 2, 2022, https://www.latimes.com/opinion/story/2022-01-02/migration-refugees-asylum-convention.

76. Médecins Sans Frontières, *Refugee Health: An Approach to Emergency Situations* (Macmillan, 1997).

77. Stephen A. Matlin, Anneliese Depoux, Stefanie Schütte, Antoine Flahault, and Luciano Saso, "Migrants' and Refugees' Health: Towards an Agenda of Solutions," *Public Health Reviews* 39, no. 1 (2018): 1–55.

78. Dinesh Bhugra, Tom Craig, and Kamaldeep Bhui, eds., *Mental Health of Refugees and Asylum Seekers* (Oxford University Press, 2010).

79. Lindsey N. Kingston, Elizabeth F. Cohen, and Christopher P. Morley, "Debate: Limitations on Universality: The 'Right to Health' and the Necessity of Legal Nationality," *BMC International Health and Human Rights* 10, no. 1 (2010): 1–12.

80. A. H. Amara and S. M. Aljunid, "Noncommunicable Diseases among Urban Refugees and Asylum-Seekers in Developing Countries: A Neglected Health Care Need," *Globalization and Health* 10, no. 1 (2014): 1–15.

81. Diane Duclos and Jennifer Palmer, "COVID-19 in the Context of Forced Displacement: Perspectives from the Middle East and East Africa," Social Science in Humanitarian Action Platform, 2020.

82. "Why It's Time to Bring Refugees Out of the Statistical Shadows," World Economic Forum, November 15, 2021, https://www.weforum.org/agenda/2021/11/refugees-internally-displaced-people-data/.

83. Heidrun Bohnet and Seraina Rüegger, "Refugees and COVID-19: Beyond Health Risks to Insecurity," *Swiss Political Science Review* 27, no. 2 (2021): 353–68.

84. "Yemen: Houthis Risk Civilians' Health in COVID-19," Human Rights Watch (website), June 1, 2021, https://www.hrw.org/news/2021/06/01/yemen-houthis-risk-civilians-health-covid-19.

85. Mohammed Alsabri, Ayman Alhadheri, Luai M. Alsakkaf, and Jennifer Cole, "Conflict and COVID-19 in Yemen: Beyond the Humanitarian Crisis," *Globalization and Health* 17, no. 1 (2021): 1–3.

86. "A Conversation with Paul Spiegel on the Afghan Healthcare System," transcript, Center for Strategic and International Studies, January 3, 2022, https://www.csis.org/analysis/conversation-paul-spiegel-afghan-healthcare-system.

87. Ángela Méndez-Triviño, "Forced Back Home by the Pandemic, Venezuelan Grandmother Sees No Choice but to Flee Once Again," UNHCR, December 10, 2020, https://www.unhcr.org/en-us/news/stories/2020/12/5fd14a064/forced-home-pandemic-venezuelan-grandmother-sees-choice-flee-once.html.

88. Zuha Siddiqui, "For Afghan Refugees, Pakistan Is a Nightmare—but Also Home," *Foreign Policy*, May 9, 2019, https://foreignpolicy.com/2019/05/09/for-afghan-refugees-pakistan-is-a-nightmare-but-also-home/.

89. Daniel A. Kronenfeld, "Afghan Refugees in Pakistan: Not All Refugees, Not Always in Pakistan, Not Necessarily Afghan?," *Journal of Refugee Studies* 21, no. 1 (2008): 43–63.

90. Lars Erslev Andersen, "The Neglected: Palestinian Refugees in Lebanon and the Syrian Refugee Crisis," Danish Institute for International Studies Report, No. 2016:12 (2016).

91. Sarah Vancluysen, "Deconstructing Borders: Mobility Strategies of South Sudanese Refugees in Northern Uganda," *Global Networks* 22, no. 1 (2022): 20–35.

92. Ryan Joseph O'Byrne and Charles Ogeno, "Pragmatic Mobilities and Uncertain Lives: Agency and the Everyday Mobility of South Sudanese Refugees in Uganda," *Journal of Refugee Studies* 33, no. 4 (2020): 747–65.

Chapter 2
The History of Forcibly Displaced Persons and Refugee Camps

1. Dimitri O'Donnell, "The Displaced and 'Forgotten' in Colombia's Soacha Slum," *Al Jazeera*, September 24, 2017, https://www.aljazeera.com/features /2017/9/24/the-displaced-and-forgotten-in-colombias-soacha-slum.

2. Michael Rummel, "Some Venezuelan Refugees Resort to Sex Work in Colombia to Survive," Voice of America, February 4, 2020, https://www .voanews.com/a/americas_some-venezuelan-refugees-resort-sex-work -colombia-survive/6183702.html.

3. Alfonso J. Rodríguez-Morales, D. Katterine Bonilla-Aldana, Miguel Morales, José A. Suárez, and Ernesto Martínez-Buitrago, "Migration Crisis in Venezuela and Its Impact on HIV in Other Countries: The Case of Colombia," *Annals of Clinical Microbiology and Antimicrobials* 18, no. 1 (2019): 1–5.

4. "Where the Streets Have No Name," *Dawn News*, December 22, 2008, https://www.dawn.com/news/434820/where-the-streets-have-no-name.

5. Irit Katz, *The Common Camp: Architecture of Power and Resistance in Israel–Palestine* (University of Minnesota Press, 2022), 2.

6. Aidan Forth, *Barbed-Wire Imperialism: Britain's Empire of Camps, 1876–1903*, Berkeley Series in British Studies, ed. Mark Bevir and James Vernon, vol. 12 (University of California Press, 2017), 223–24.

7. Benjamin Thomas White, "Humans and Animals in a Refugee Camp: Baquba, Iraq, 1918–20," *Journal of Refugee Studies* 32, no. 2 (2019): 216–36.

8. Laura Robson, "Refugee Camps and the Spatialization of Assyrian Nationalism in Iraq," in *Modernity, Minority, and the Public Sphere*, ed. S. R. Goldstein-Sabbah and H. L. Murre-van den Berg (Brill, 2016), 237–57.

9. Baher Ibrahim, "Refugee Settlement and Encampment in the Middle East and North Africa, 1860s–1940s," research guide, 2021, https://static1 .squarespace.com/static/5748678dcf80a1ffcaf26975/t/614ca66b 9294e2269debb27a/1632413293154/.

10. White, "Humans and Animals."

11. Louise W. Holborn, "The League of Nations and the Refugee Problem," *Annals of the American Academy of Political and Social Science* 203, no. 1 (1939): 124–35.

12. Mira L. Siegelberg, "Statelessness," in *Statelessness: A Modern History*, by Mira L. Siegelberg (Harvard University Press, 2020).

13. Bruno Cabanes, *The Great War and the Origins of Humanitarianism, 1918–1924* (Cambridge University Press, 2014), 133–39.

14. Ariadna Tyrkova-Williams, December 1921, British Library, Tyrkova-Williams Collection, Add MS 54466, ff. 93–96; see "The Russian Refugee Crisis of the 1920s," British Library's European Studies Blog, December 10, 2015, https://blogs.bl.uk/european/2015/12/the-russian -refugee-crisis-of-the-1920s.html.

15. The Record of the Save the Children Fund, December 15, 1921, p. 107, Cadbury Research Library, Special Collections, SCF Box A670, University of Birmingham.

16. Cabanes, *The Great War*, 135–37.

17. Cabanes, *The Great War*, 140–43.

18. Nicola Migliorino, *(Re)constructing Armenia in Lebanon and Syria: Ethno-cultural Diversity and the State in the Aftermath of a Refugee Crisis*, Forced Migration, vol. 21 (Berghahn Books, 2008), 30–31.

19. Mark R. Baker, "The Armenian Genocide and Its Denial: A Review of Recent Scholarship," *New Perspectives on Turkey* 53 (2015): 197–212.

20. For a history of the League of Nations, see: Ruth Henig, *The Peace That Never Was: A History of the League of Nations* (Haus Publishing, 2019); and Martyn Housden, *The League of Nations and the Organization of Peace* (Routledge, 2014).

21. Siegelberg, "Statelessness," 51–57.

22. For a detailed biography of Nansen, see Roland Huntford, *Nansen: The Explorer as Hero* (Abacus, 2012).

23. D'Arcy W. Thompson, "Fridtjof Nansen: 10 October 1861–13 May 1930," *ICES Journal of Marine Science* 5, no. 2 (August 1930): 141–48.

24. For details on the trip, see: Fridjtof Nansen, *Farthest North: The Incredible Three-Year Voyage to the Frozen Latitudes of the North* (Modern Library, 2000).
25. Fridtjof Nansen and S. Kjærheim, *Fridtjof Nansen* (Berliner Illustrations-Gesellschaft, 1905).
26. Cabanes, *The Great War*, 155.
27. Vincent Chetail, "Fridtjof Nansen and the International Protection of Refugees: An Introduction," *Refugee Survey Quarterly* 22, no. 1 (2003): 1–6.
28. Jon Sorenson, *The Saga of Fridtjof Nansen* (Allen and Unwin, 1932), 270.
29. Huntford, *Nansen*, 442–43.
30. Hannah Astrup Larsen, "Pity and Charity: Nansen's Cure for World Misery," *New York Times*, October 28, 1923.
31. Cabanes, *The Great War*, 156–64.
32. Cabanes, The Great War, 156–64.
33. Cabanes, The Great War, 156–64.
34. Cabanes, *The Great War*, 162.
35. M. Fosse and J. Fox, *Nansen: Explorer and Humanitarian* (Rowman & Littlefield, 2015), 56–64.
36. Martyn Housden, "White Russians Crossing the Black Sea: Fridtjof Nansen, Constantinople and the First Modern Repatriation of Refugees Displaced by Civil Conflict, 1922–23," *Slavonic and East European Review* 88, no. 3 (2010): 495–524.
37. Cabanes, *The Great War*, 162.
38. Cabanes, *The Great War*, 164.
39. See Otto Hieronymi, "The Nansen Passport: A Tool of Freedom of Movement and of Protection," *Refugee Survey Quarterly* 22, no. 1 (2003): 36–47; and Peter Gatrell, "The Nansen Passport: The Innovative Response to the Refugee Crisis That Followed the Russian Revolution," *The Conversation*, November 6, 2017, http://theconversation. com /thenansen-passport-the-innovative-response-to-the-refugee-crisis-that -followed-the-russian-revolution-85487.
40. Louise W. Holborn, "The Legal Status of Political Refugees, 1920–1938," *American Journal of International Law* 32, no. 4 (1938): 680–703.
41. Gatrell, "The Nansen Passport."
42. Cabanes, *The Great War*, 164–73.

43. George Ginsburgs, "The Soviet Union and the Problem of Refugees and Displaced Persons 1917–1956," *American Journal of International Law* 51, no. 2 (1957): 325–61.

44. Cabanes, *The Great War*, 170.

45. Colin Jones, Paul Weindling, and Charles Rosenberg, eds., *International Health Organisations and Movements*, 1918–1939 (Cambridge University Press, 1995).

46. Jones et al., *International Health Organisations*, 96–102.

47. Paul Weindling, Roger Cooter, and John Pickstone, "Health and Medicine in Interwar Europe," in *Companion to Medicine in the Twentieth Century*, ed. Roger Cooter and John Pickstone (Taylor & Francis, 2003), 39–50.

48. Francis Cox, "The First World War: Disease, The Only Victor," lecture, Gresham College, March 10, 2014, https://www.gresham.ac.uk/watch -now/first-world-war-disease-only-victor.

49. K. David Patterson and Gerald F. Pyle, "The Geography and Mortality of the 1918 Influenza Pandemic," *Bulletin of the History of Medicine* 65, no. 1 (1991): 4–21.

50. David P. Forsythe, *The Humanitarians: The International Committee of the Red Cross* (Cambridge University Press, 2005), 29–38.

51. Walter Ewing, "Opportunity and Exclusion: A Brief History of US Immigration Policy," Immigration Policy Center, American Immigration Council, January 2012, https://www.americanimmigrationcouncil.org /research/opportunity-and-exclusion-brief-history-us-immigration-policy.

52. Ross Laurie, "Reporting on Race: White Australia, Immigration and the Popular Press in the 1920s," *Journal of the Royal Historical Society of Queensland* 18, no. 10 (2004): 420–31.

53. Leo Lucassen, "The Great War and the Origins of Migration Control in Western Europe and the United States (1880–1920)," in *Regulation of Migration: International Experiences*, ed. Anita Böcker, Kees Groe- nendijk, Tetty Havinga, Paul Minderhaud (Het Spinhuis, 1998): 45–72.

54. For an excellent analysis, see Keith David Watenpaugh, *Bread from Stones: The Middle East and the Making of Modern Humanitarianism* (University of California Press, 2015).

55. Philippe Bourmaud, "Between Nationalism, Internationalism and Colonial Quadrillage: The Action Chrétienne en Orient in Mandatory Syria (1922–1946)," *Transformation* 39, no. 1 (2022): 30–44.

56. For a history of Save the Children, see: Emily Baughan, *Saving the Children: Humanitarianism, Internationalism, and Empire*, Berkeley Series in British Studies, vol. 19 (University of California Press, 2021).

57. Jean Allman, "Making Mothers: Missionaries, Medical Officers and Women's Work in Colonial Asante, 1924–1945," *History Workshop Journal*, vol. 38, no. 1 (1994): 23–47.

58. See Katz, *Common Camp*, 1–9.

59. Watenpaugh, *Bread from Stones*, 176.

60. Benjamin Thomas White, "Humans and Animals in Refugee Camps, Past and Present, Refugee History (website), June 2018, http://refugeehistory .org/blog/2018/6/21/humans-and-animals-in-refugee-camps-past-and -present.

61. Marvin Kalb, "Refugee Crises and the Sad Legacy of the 1938 Evian Conference," Brookings (website), September 23, 2015.

62. Neil Smith, *American Empire* (University of California Press, 2003), 295.

63. Laura Robson, "What Are Refugee Camps For?," *Current Affairs*, January 7, 2020.

64. Earl G. Harrison, Report, 1945, https://www.eisenhowerlibrary.gov/sites /default/files/research/online-documents/holocaust/report-harrison.pdf.

65. Riccardo Bocco, "UNRWA and the Palestinian Refugees: A History within History," *Refugee Survey Quarterly* 28, no. 2–3 (2009): 229–52.

66. Susan Akram, *UNRWA and Palestinian Refugees* (Oxford University Press, 2014).

67. Elena Fiddian-Qasmiyeh, "The Changing Faces of UNRWA: From the Global to the Local," *Journal of Humanitarian Affairs* 1, no. 1 (2019): 28–41.

68. Peter Beaumont and Oliver Holmes, "US Confirms End to Funding for UN Palestinian Refugees," *Guardian*, August 31, 2018, https://www .theguardian.com/world/2018/aug/31/trump-to-cut-all-us-funding-for -uns-main-palestinian-refugee-programme.

69. For details on the origin of UNHCR, power struggle, and East-West tension, see: Gil Loescher, *The UNHCR and World Politics: A Perilous Path* (Oxford University Press, 2001), 34–46.

70. The rule of the British was called *the British Raj*; the term *Raj* in Hindi and in Urdu means to rule.

71. V. F. Y. Zamindar, *The Long Partition and the Making of Modern South Asia: Refugees, Boundaries, Histories* (Columbia University Press, 2007).

72. William Henderson, "The Refugees in India and Pakistan," *Journal of International Affairs* (1953): 57–65.

73. Elisabetta Iob, *Refugees and the Politics of the Everyday State in Pakistan: Resettlement in Punjab, 1947–1962* (Routledge, 2017).

74. Ian Talbot, "Pakistan: Refugee State," in *Refugee Crises, 1945–2000: Political and Societal Responses in International Comparison*, ed. Jan C. Jansen and Simone Lässig (Cambridge University Press, 2020), 83–103.

75. See, for example: "10,000 Muslim Refugees Arrive in Lahore from Beas on October 8," *Pakistan Times*, October 10, 1947, p. 3; and "50,000 Refugees Enter Pakistan on October 22," *Pakistan Times*, October 23, 1947.

76. Muhammad H. Zaman, "Transitional Statelessness: Drugs, Disease, and Denial of Refugee Care in the New State of Pakistan," Stateless Histories (website), Pennsylvania State University, January 24, 2022, https:// statelesshistories.org/article/transitional-statelessness-and-its -consequences-drugs-disease-and-denial-of-care-for-refugees-in-the-new -state-of-pakistan.

77. Zaman, "Transitional Statelessness."

78. Iob, *Refugees and the Politics of the Everyday State*, 46.

79. For most of the fall of 1947, a weekly section called "Refugee Corner" appeared in major Pakistani newspapers that described the plight of the refugees.

80. Deputy High Commissioner Lahore Report, August 27, 1948, DO 142/440, Refugees in West Punjab, National Archives, Kew.

81. There is a whole genre in Urdu fiction called *Taqsim ka adab* (literature of partition) that was often banned and viewed as either too raw, too vulgar, anti-Islamic, or anti-state.

82. For a description of the Citizen's Archive of Pakistan (Oral History Project), see: https://participedia.net/case/4548.

83. Jehan Ul Mulk, Basit Ali, and Atta Ullah, "Impacts of Afghan Refugees on Security Situation of Pakistan," *Pakistan Journal of Society, Education and Language* 6, no. 1 (2020): 37–46.

84. "A Refugee Camp Becomes a City," *Living on Earth* (radio news magazine), May 3, 2019, https://www.loe.org/shows/segments.html ?programID=19-P13-00018&segmentID=1.

85. Ben Rawlence, *City of Thorns: Nine Lives in the World's Largest Refugee Camp* (Picador, 2016).

86. Shayaan Subzwari, "Sanitation and Water Access for Pakistan's Afghan Refugees," January 18, 2021, Paani (website), https://www.paaniproject .org/sanitation-and-water-access-for-pakistans-afghan-refugees/.

87. Sean Anderson and Jennifer Ferng, "The Detention-Industrial Complex in Australia," *Journal of the Society of Architectural Historians* 73, no. 4 (2014): 469–74.

88. Robson, "What Are Refugee Camps For?"

89. For recent literature see: Irit Katz, Diana Martín, and Claudio Minca, eds., *Camps Revisited: Multifaceted Spatialities of a Modern Political Technology* (Rowman & Littlefield, 2018); and Tom Scott-Smith and Mark E. Breeze, eds. *Structures of Protection? Rethinking Refugee Shelter,* Forced Migration, vol. 39 (Berghahn Books, 2020).

90. Romola Sanyal, "A No-Camp Policy: Interrogating Informal Settlements in Lebanon," *Geoforum* 84 (2017): 117–25.

91. Romola Sanyal, "Refugees and the City: An Urban Discussion," *Geography Compass* 6, no. 11 (2012): 633–44.

92. Robson, "What Are Refugee Camps For?"

93. Lee W. Riley, Albert I. Ko, Alon Unger, and Mitermayer G. Reis, "Slum Health: Diseases of Neglected Populations," *BMC International Health and Human Rights* 7, no. 1 (2007): 1–6.

94. Jobair Alam, "The Status and Rights of the Rohingya as Refugees under International Refugee Law: Challenges for a Durable Solution," *Journal of Immigrant & Refugee Studies* 19, no. 2 (2021): 128–41.

95. Jean Pierre Maniraguha, "Challenges of Reintegrating Returning Refugees: A Case study of Returnee Access to Land and to Basic Services in Burundi" (master's thesis, Universitetet i Tromsø, 2011).

96. Heidrun Bohnet, "Back to Turmoil: Refugee and IDP Return to and within South Sudan," Bonn International Center for Conversion working paper, 2016, 37, https://www.ssoar.info/ssoar/handle/document /61659.

97. Catherine Huser, Andrew Cunningham, Christine Kamau, and Mary Obara, "South Sudanese Returns: Perceptions and Responses," *Forced Migration Review* 62 (2019): 7–10.

98. Sarah Vancluysen, "Deconstructing Borders: Mobility Strategies of South Sudanese Refugees in Northern Uganda," *Global Networks* 22, no. 1 (2022): 20–35.

99. Giulio Coppi, *The Humanitarian Crisis in Yemen: Beyond the Man-Made Disaster* (International Peace Institute, 2018).

100. Stean Auguste Tshiband, "Breaking the Vicious Circle: Exploring Alternatives to Current Responses and Solutions to Internal Displacement in Yemen," London School of Economics and Political Science's Middle East Centre Blog, February 16, 2018, https://blogs.lse.ac.uk/mec /2018/02/16/breaking-the-vicious-circle-exploring-alternatives-to -current-responses-and-solutions-to-internal-displacement-in-yemen/.

101. Peter Heudtlass, Niko Speybroeck, and Debarati Guha-Sapir, "Excess Mortality in Refugees, Internally Displaced Persons and Resident Populations in Complex Humanitarian Emergencies (1998–2012): Insights from Operational Data," *Conflict and Health* 10, no. 1 (2016): 1–11.

102. Firdausi Qadri, Taufiqul Islam, and John D. Clemens, "Cholera in Yemen—An Old Foe Rearing Its Ugly Head," *New England Journal of Medicine* 377, no. 21 (2017): 2005–7.

103. "Yemen: Mobile Clinics Make Medical Care Possible amid the Crisis," Relief Web (website), November 18, 2021, https://reliefweb.int/report /yemen/yemen-mobile-clinics-make-medical-care-possible-amid-crisis.

104. Sara Jerving, "Yemen's Health System Is Hanging 'On a Cliff,'" Devex (website), February 17, 2022, https://www.devex.com/news/yemen-s -health-system-is-hanging-on-a-cliff-102543.

105. Mohammed Alshakka, Mohamed Izham Mohamed Ibrahim, Awsan Bahattab, Wafa F. S. Badulla, and P. Ravi Shankar, "An Insight into the Pharmaceutical Sector in Yemen during Conflict: Challenges and Recommendations," *Medicine, Conflict and Survival* 36, no. 3 (2020): 232–48.

106. "UnSettlement: Urban Displacement in the 21st Century" (Internal Displacement Monitoring Center, 2018), https://www.internal-displacement .org/publications/unsettlement-urban-displacement-in-the-21st-century.

107. "Additional Provisions within the Revised National Refugee Law in Ethiopia," UNHCR report, (undated), https://data.unhcr.org/en /documents/download/68014.

Chapter 3
Models of Health Care Systems

1. Vivian Sequera and Francisco Aguilar, "As Economic Crisis Worsens, Schools Empty in Venezuela, *Christian Science Monitor*, April 25, 2018,

https://www.csmonitor.com/World/Americas/2018/0425/As-economic-crisis-worsens-schools-empty-in-Venezuela.

2. Juan Manuel Rodríguez Vargas, Eunice Danitza Vargas Valle, and Ana María López Jaramillo, "The Affiliation to the Health System among Venezuelan Migrants in Colombia," *Población y Salud en Mesoamérica* 18, no. 2 (2021): 181–214.

3. Muhammad Hamid Zaman, Tahera Hasan, and Janki Bhatt, "Invisible People, Visible Barriers: Healthcare Access for and among Ethnic Bengalis in Pakistan," *Statelessness & Citizenship Review* 4, no. 2 (2022): 286–92, https://statelessnessandcitizenshipreview.com/index.php/journal/article/view/357.

4. Alizeh Kohari, "Marooned: Karachi's Stateless Fishermen," November 3, 2021, Coda Story (website), https://www.codastory.com/authoritarian-tech/bengali-pakistan-nadra-biometrics/.

5. Maheen Nisar, Rubaab M. Mohammad, Sani Fatima, Preet R. Shaikh, and Mehroze Rehman, "Perceptions Pertaining to Clinical Depression in Karachi, Pakistan," *Cureus* 11, no. 7 (2019).

6. Elizabeth A. Rowley, Gilbert M. Burnham, and Rabbin M. Drabe. "Protracted Refugee Situations: Parallel Health Systems and Planning for the Integration off Services," *Journal of Refugee Studies* 19, no. 2 (2006): 158–86.

7. World Health Organization, "Mapping Health Systems' Responsiveness to Refugee and Migrant Health Needs," October 19, 2021, https://www.who.int/publications/i/item/9789240030640.

8. Maureen Mackintosh, Amos Channon, Anup Karan, Sakthivel Selvaraj, Eleonora Cavagnero, and Hongwen Zhao, "What is the Private Sector? Understanding Private Provision in the Health Systems of Low-Income and Middle-Income Countries," *Lancet* 388, no. 10044 (2016): 596–605; Anne Mills, "Health Care Systems in Low- and Middle-income Countries," *New England Journal of Medicine* 370, no. 6 (2014): 552–57.

9. For example, see: Murad Moosa Khan, "Private Healthcare in Pakistan—Costly, Unregulated and Predatory, *Express Tribune*, November 18, 2019, https://tribune.com.pk/article/90951/private-healthcare-in-pakistan-costly-unregulated-and-predatory.

10. W. de St. Aubin, "Peace and Refugees in the Middle East," *Middle East Journal* (1949): 249–59.

11. Colin Jones, Paul Weindling, and Charles Rosenberg, eds., *International Health Organisations and Movements, 1918–1939* (Cambridge University Press, 1995).

12. Kirsten McConnachie, "Camps of Containment: A Genealogy of the Refugee Camp," *Humanity: An International Journal of Human Rights, Humanitarianism, and Development* 7, no. 3 (2016): 397–412.

13. Inger Marie Okkenhaug and Karène Sanchez Summerer, *Christian Missions and Humanitarianism in the Middle East, 1850–1950: Ideologies, Rhetoric, and Practices* (Brill, 2020).

14. Linnea Patterson, "Diseases in Refugee Camps: What We Can Learn from 1947," 1947 Partition Archive, September 24, 2020, https://www.1947partitionarchive.org/disease_and_Partition.

15. Beryl Cheal, "Refugees in the Gaza Strip, December 1948–May 1950," *Journal of Palestine Studies* 18, no. 1 (1988): 138–57.

16. W. Pieper and U. L. Jentz, "A Typhoid Epidemic in a Refugee Camp," *Archiv für Hygiene und Bakteriolgie* 133, no. 4 (1950): 271–84.

17. Paula E. Brentlinger, "Health, Human Rights, and Malaria Control: Historical Background and Current Challenges," *Health and Human Rights* (2006): 10–38; and Swati Sengupta Chatterjee, "Sanitation and Health at West Bengal Refugee Camps in the 1950s," *Vidyasagar University Journal of History* 3 (2014–2015): 82–94.

18. Elisabetta Iob, *Refugees and the Politics of the Everyday State in Pakistan: Resettlement in Punjab, 1947–1962* (Routledge, 2017), 46–51.

19. Iob, *Refugees and the Politics of the Everday State.*

20. Iob, *Refugees and the Politics of the Everday State.*

21. Muhammad H. Zaman, "Transitional Statelessness: Drugs, Disease, and Denial of Refugee Care in the New State of Pakistan," Stateless Histories (website), Pennsylvania State University, January 24, 2022, https://statelesshistories.org/article/transitional-statelessness-and-its-consequences-drugs-disease-and-denial-of-care-for-refugees-in-the-new-state-of-pakistan.

22. Julia R. Shatz, "A Politics of Care: Local Nurses in Mandate Palestine," *International Journal of Middle East Studies* 50, no. 4 (2018): 669–89.

23. Mihoko Tanabe, Anna Myers, Prem Bhandari, Nadine Cornier, Sathyanarayanan Doraiswamy, and Sandra Krause, "Family Planning in Refugee

Settings: Findings and Actions from a Multi-Country Study," *Conflict and Health* 11, no. 1 (2017): 1–12.

24. Shadi Saleh, Sarah Ibrahim, Jasmin Lilian Diab, and Mona Osman, "Integrating Refugees into National Health Systems amid Political and Economic Constraints in the EMR: Approaches from Lebanon and Jordan," *Journal of Global Health* 12 (2022).

25. "Employment of Palestine Refugees in Lebanon: An Overview," UNRWA for Palestine Refugees in the Near East, May 23, 2016, https://www.unrwa.org/resources/reports/employment-palestine-refugees-lebanon-overview.

26. Jad Chaaban, Hala Ghattas, Rima Habib, Sari Hanafi, Nadine Sahyoun, Nisreen Salti, Karin Seyfert, and Nadia Naamani, "Socio-economic Survey of Palestinian Refugees in Lebanon," report published by the American University of Beirut and the UNRWA for Palestine Refugees in the Near East, 2010, https://www.unrwa.org/resources/reports/socio-economic-survey-palestinian-refugees-lebanon.

27. Lina Abu-Habib, "Education and the Palestinian Refugees of Lebanon: A Lost Generation," *Refugee Participation Network* 21 (1996): 94–111.

28. Lama Al-Arian, "In Lebanon, Palestinians Protest New Employment Restrictions, NPR, July 26, 2019, https://www.npr.org/2019/07/26/745041157/in-lebanon-palestinians-protest-new-employment-restrictions.

29. U. Krause, *Difficult Life in a Refugee Camp: Gender, Violence, and Coping in Uganda* (Cambridge University Press, 2021), 90–145.

30. Eve Lester, "A Place at the Table: The Role of NGOs in Refugee Protection: International Advocacy and Policy-making," *Refugee Survey Quarterly* 24, no. 2 (2005): 125–42.

31. Dina Zyadeh, "Developing Humanitarian Innovation Impact Metrics: Where Do We Start?," UNHCR (website), https://www.unhcr.org/innovation/developing-humanitarian-innovation-impact-metrics-start/.

32. David Keen, *Complex Emergencies* (Polity, 2008), 157.

33. Keen, *Complex Emergencies*, 157.

34. Jeff Crisp and Karen Jacobsen, "Refugee Camps Reconsidered," *Forced Migration Review* 3, no. 12 (1998): 27–30.

35. Philippe Goyens, Denis Porignon, Entienne Mugisho Soron'gane, and Rene Tonglet, "Humanitarian Aid and Health Services in Eastern Kivu, Zaire: Collaboration or Competition," *Journal of Refugee Studies* 9 (1996): 268.

36. Simon Turner, "What Is a Refugee Camp? Explorations of the Limits and Effects of the Camp," *Journal of Refugee Studies* 29, no. 2 (2016): 139–48.
37. Stephen A. Matlin, Anneliese Depoux, Stefanie Schütte, Antoine Flahault, and Luciano Saso, "Migrants' and Refugees' Health: Towards an Agenda of Solutions," *Public Health Reviews* 39, no. 1 (2018): 1–55.
38. Matlin et. al, "Migrants' and Refugees' Health."
39. Egbert Sondorp, Tania Kaiser, and Anthony Zwi, "Beyond Emergency Care: Challenges to Health Planning in Complex Emergencies," *Tropical Medicine & International Health* 6, no. 12 (2001): 965–70.
40. Anupama Thiagarajan and Maria Syed, "Refugee Camps: The Informal Permanence of Temporary Infrastructure," *CRIT* [journal of the American Institute of Architecture Students] 82 (2018): 19–20.
41. Fayez Azez Mahamid, "Collective Trauma, Quality of Life and Resilience in Narratives of Third-Generation Palestinian Refugee Children," *Child Indicators Research* 13, no. 6 (2020): 2181–204.
42. Ilana Feldman, "Humanitarian Care and the Ends of Life: The Politics of Aging and Dying in a Palestinian Refugee Camp," *Cultural Anthropology* 32, no. 1 (2017): 42–67.
43. Isabel Pinheiro and Dilshad Jaff, "The Role of Palliative Care in Addressing the Health Needs of Syrian Refugees in Jordan," *Medicine, Conflict and Survival* 34, no. 1 (2018): 19–38.
44. M. Mahruf C. Shohel, "Education in Emergencies: Challenges of Providing Education for Rohingya Children Living in Refugee Camps in Bangladesh," *Education Inquiry* 13, no. 1 (2022): 104–26.
45. Tony Waters and Kim LeBlanc, "Refugees and Education: Mass Public Schooling without a Nation-state," *Comparative Education Review* 49, no. 2 (2005): 129–47.
46. Najwa Rizkallah, "Nutritional Status of Primary School Children in a Refugee Camp of the West Bank" (Institute of Community and Public Health, Birzeit University, 1991).
47. Farshad Rastegar, "Education and Revolutionary Political Mobilization: Schooling versus Uprootedness as Determinants of Islamic Political Activism among Afghan Refugee Students in Pakistan" (PhD diss., University of California, Los Angeles, 1991).
48. Shelly Culbertson and Louay Constant, "Education of Syrian Refugee Children: Managing the Crisis in Turkey, Lebanon, and Jordan" (Santa Monica, CA: RAND Corp., 2015).

49. Mehreen Usman, "Afghan Diaspora in Pakistan: Health and Education Policy Recommendations for Rural and Urban Areas," Refugee Research Online (website), January 6, 2020, https://refugeeresearchonline.org /afghan-diaspora-in-pakistan-healthcare-and-education-policy -recommendations/.

50. Hiba Salem, "Realities of School 'Integration': Insights from Syrian Refugee Students in Jordan's Double-shift Schools," *Journal of Refugee Studies* 34, no. 4 (2022): 4188–206.

51. Julia Mahfouz, Nizar El-Mehtar, Enja Osman, and Stephen Kotok, "Challenges and Agency: Principals Responding to the Syrian Refugee Crisis in Lebanese Public Schools," *International Journal of Leadership in Education* (2019).

52. Anais Tuepker and Chunhuei Chi, "Evaluating Integrated Healthcare for Refugees and Hosts in an African Context," *Health Economics, Policy and Law* 4, no. 2 (2009): 159–78.

53. For a detailed analysis of this complex relationship, see Kelsey P. Norman, *Reluctant Reception: Refugees, Migration and Governance in the Middle East and North Africa* (Cambridge University Press, 2020).

54. Anna Getmansky, Tolga Sınmazdemir, and Thomas Zeitzoff, "Refugees, Xenophobia, and Domestic Conflict: Evidence from a Survey Experiment in Turkey," *Journal of Peace Research* 55, no. 4 (2018): 491–507.

55. Savannah Cellocco, Rizwan Khan, Brunilda Elezi, and Giulia Carpineti, "The Afghanistan-Pakistan Case: A Reverse Exodus of Afghan Refugees," Università di Macerata, 2018.

56. Fatina Abreek-Zubiedat and Alona Nitzan-Shiftan, "'De-Camping' through Development: The Palestinian Refugee Camps in the Gaza Strip under the Israeli Occupation," in *Camps Revisited: Multifaceted Spatialities of a Modern Political Technology*, by Irit Katz, Diana Martin, and Claudio Minca (Rowman & Littlefield, 2018), 137–57.

57. Zia ur-Rehman, "Afghans Flee to Pakistan: An Uncertain Future Awaits," *New York Times*, September 8, 2021, https://www.nytimes.com/2021/09 /08/world/asia/pakistan-afghanistan-refugees.html.

58. Rebecca Shaeffer, "No Healing Here: Violence, Discrimination and Barriers to Health for Migrants in South Africa," Human Rights Watch (website), December 7, 2009, https://www.hrw.org/report/2009/12/07 /no-healing-here/violence-discrimination-and-barriers-health-migrants -south-africa.

59. Several recent Twitter campaigns in Pakistan have used hashtags like *Namakharam* (a derogatory term meaning ungrateful) regarding Afghan refugees.

60. Mike Berry, Iñaki Garcia-Blanco, and Kerry Moore, "Press Coverage of the Refugee and Migrant Crisis in the EU: A Content Analysis of Five European Countries," report prepared for UNHCR, Cardiff School of Journalism, Media and Cultural Studies, 2016, http://www.unhcr.org/56bb369c9.html.

61. Jonathan Crush and Godfrey Tawodzera, "Medical Xenophobia and Zimbabwean Migrant Access to Public Health Services in South Africa," *Journal of Ethnic and Migration Studies* 40, no. 4 (2014): 655–70.

62. Personal communication with public hospital administrators in Karachi, Pakistan, 2019 and 2020.

63. Brennan Hoban, "Do Immigrants 'Steal' Jobs from American Workers?," Brookings (website), August 24, 2017, https://www.brookings.edu/blog/brookings-now/2017/08/24/do-immigrants-steal-jobs-from-american-workers/.

64. Christopher Garimoi Orach and Vincent De Brouwere, "Integrating Refugee and Host Health Services in West Nile Districts, Uganda," *Health Policy and Planning* 21, no. 1 (2006): 53–64.

65. Lara Alshawawreh, "Architecture of Emergencies in The Middle East: Proposed Shelter Design Criteria" (PhD diss., Edinburgh Napier University, 2019).

66. E. Sukkar, "Supplying Medicines to Refugees: A Logistical Nightmare," *Pharmaceutical Journal* 294, no. 7851 (2015).

67. Alexandra Francis, "Jordan's Refugee Crisis," Carnegie Endowment for International Peace (website), September 21, 2015, https://carnegieendowment.org/2015/09/21/jordan-s-refugee-crisis-pub-61338.

68. Saleh et al., "Integrating Refugees into National Health Systems."

69. Naseeb Qirbi and Sharif A. Ismail, "Health System Functionality in a Low-income Country in the Midst of Conflict: The Case of Yemen," *Health Policy and Planning* 32, no. 6 (2017): 911–22.

70. Shannon Doocy, Emily Lyles, Laila Akhu-Zaheya, Ann Burton, and Gilbert Burnham, "Health Service Access and Utilization among Syrian Refugees in Jordan," *International Journal for Equity in Health* 15, no. 1 (2016): 1–15.

71. Carolyn L. Tobin, Pam Di Napoli, and Cheryl Tatano Beck, "Refugee and Immigrant Women's Experience of Postpartum Depression: A

Meta-Synthesis," *Journal of Transcultural Nursing* 29, no. 1 (2018): 84–100.

72. Diana Martin and Julia Brown, "'Littered with Logos!': An Investigation into the Relationship between Water Provision, Humanitarian Branding, Donor Accountability, and Self-Reliance in Ugandan Refugee Settlements," *Refugee Survey Quarterly* 40, no. 4 (2021): 433–58.

73. World Health Organization, "Health Promotion for Improved Refugee and Migrant Health: Technical Guidance," 2018, https://apps.who.int /iris/handle/10665/342287.

74. Assad Hafeez, Rubina Riaz, Samin Ullah Shah, Javed Pervaiz, and David Southall, "Integrating Health Care for Mothers and Children in Refugee Camps and at District Level," *British Medical Journal* 328, no. 7443 (2004): 834–36.

75. See, for example, "Mamdot Resigns from Joint Refugee Council," *Pakistan Times*, March 26, 1948.

76. D. F. Karaka, *Freedom Must Not Stink* (Punjab: Kutub Publishers, 1947), 1, 15–16, 21.

77. Theron H. Butterworth, "Health Education for Palestine Arab Refugees," *Public Health Reports* 70, no. 10 (1955): 1011.

78. Zaman, "Transitional Statelessness." See also: Pippa Virdee, "Remembering Partition: Women, Oral Histories and the Partition of 1947," *Oral History* (2013): 49–62.

79. Joel D. Howell, "Reflections on the Past and Future of Primary Care," *Health Affairs* 29, no. 5 (2010): 760–65.

80. World Health Organization, "Minutes of the Second Meeting: Held at the Regional Office, Alexandria on Tuesday, 7 October 1969," Document No. EM/RC19A/Min.2, https://apps.who.int/iris/handle/10665 /124356.

81. P. Garner, Trudy Harpham, and Hugh Annett, "Information Support for Urban Primary Health Care," *World Health Forum* 13, no. 2/3 (1992): 244–49.

82. "MSF Opens New Clinic in Karachi, Pakistan's Largest City," Médecins Sans Frontières, December 27, 2012, https://www.doctorswithoutborders .org/latest/msf-opens-new-clinic-karachi-pakistans-largest-city.

83. Harriet Blundell, Rachael Milligan, Susan L. Norris, and Paul Garner, "WHO Guidance for Refugees in Camps: Systematic Review," *BMJ Open* 9, no. 9 (2019): e027094.

84. Tala Al-Rousan, Zaker Schwabkey, Lara Jirmanus, and Brett D. Nelson, "Health Needs and Priorities of Syrian Refugees in Camps and Urban Settings in Jordan: Perspectives of Refugees and Health Care Providers," *Eastern Mediterranean Health Journal* 24, no. 3 (2018): 243–53.

85. Dilaver Tengilimoğlu, Aysu Zekioğlu, Fatih Budak, Hüseyin Eriş, and Mustafa Younis, "Refugees' Opinions about Healthcare Services: A Case of Turkey," *Healthcare* 9, no. 5 (2021): 490.

86. Eileen Pittaway and Linda Bartolomei, "Refugees, Race, and Gender: The Multiple Discrimination against Refugee Women," *Refuge* 19, no. 6 (2000): 21.

87. Hanina Abi Nader and William Watfa, "Why Be a Refugee Camp Doctor: The Challenges, Rewards and Medical Education Aspects," *International Journal of Medical Education* 8 (2017): 307.

88. Arwa Mahdawi, "A Doctor's Story: Inside the 'Living Hell' of Moria Refugee Camp," *Guardian*, February 9, 2020, https://www.theguardian.com /world/2020/feb/09/moria-refugee-camp-doctors-story-lesbos-greece.

89. Hannah Tappis, Sarah Elaraby, Shatha Elnakib, Nagiba A. Abdulghani AlShawafi, Huda BaSaleem, Iman Ahmed Saleh Al-Gawfi, Fouad Othman, Fouzia Shafique et al., "Reproductive, Maternal, Newborn and Child Health Service Delivery during Conflict in Yemen: A Case Study," *Conflict and Health* 14, no. 1 (2020): 1–16.

90. Boshra Alhomaide, "Displaced Yemenis Grow Desperate in Camps," Al-Monitor (website), May 31, 2022, https://www.al-monitor.com /originals/2022/05/displaced-yemenis-grow-desperate-camps.

91. Sara Jerving, "Yemen's Health System Is Hanging 'on a Cliff,'" Devex (website), February 17, 2022, https://www.devex.com/news/yemen-s -health-system-is-hanging-on-a-cliff-102543.

92. Personal communication with clinicians at the primary care clinic in Machar Colony.

93. Sandra Krause, Holly Williams, Monica A. Onyango, Samira Sami, Wilma Doedens, Noreen Giga, Erin Stone, and Barbara Tomczyk, "Reproductive Health Services for Syrian Refugees in Zaatri Camp and Irbid City, Hashemite Kingdom of Jordan: An Evaluation of the Minimum Initial Services Package," *Conflict and Health* 9, no. 1 (2015): 1–10.

94. Peter N. Fonjungo, Yenew Kebede, Tsehaynesh Messele, Gonfa Ayana, Gudeta Tibesso, Almaz Abebe, John N. Nkengasong, and Thomas Kenyon, "Laboratory Equipment Maintenance: A Critical Bottleneck for

Strengthening Health Systems in Sub-Saharan Africa?," *Journal of Public Health Policy* 33, no. 1 (2012): 34–45.

95. Elizabeth A. Rowley, Gilbert M. Burnham, and Rabbin M. Drabe, "Protracted Refugee Situations: Parallel Health Systems and Planning for the Integration of Services," *Journal of Refugee Studies* 19, no. 2 (2006): 158–86.

96. Ansbro, Éimhín, Sylvia Garry, Veena Karir, Amulya Reddy, Kiran Jobanputra, Taissir Fardous, and Zia Sadique, "Delivering a Primary-Level Non-communicable Disease Programme for Syrian Refugees and the Host Population in Jordan: A Descriptive Costing Study," *Health Policy and Planning* 35, no. 8 (2020): 931–40.

97. Daniel R. Lustick and Muhammad H. Zaman, "Biomedical Engineering Education and Practice Challenges and Opportunities in Improving Health in Developing Countries," Atlanta Conference on Science and Innovation Policy, IEEE, 2011, https://www.researchgate.net/publication/260737001 _Biomedical_engineering_education_and_practice_challenges_and _opportunities_in_improving_health_in_developing_countries.

98. "Women's Health Services Lacking for Syrian Refugees," report from Syrian American Medical Society, February 14, 2019, https://www.sams-usa.net /2019/02/14/womens-health-services-lacking-for-syrian-refugees/.

99. World Health Organization, "Improving the Health Care of Pregnant Refugee and Migrant Women and Newborn Children: Technical Guidance," 2018, https://apps.who.int/iris/handle/10665/342289.

100. Lorraine Charles and Kate Denman, "Syrian and Palestinian Syrian Refugees in Lebanon: The Plight of Women and Children," *Journal of International Women's Studies* 14, no. 5 (2013): 96–111.

101. Hawa-Idil Harakow, Lone Hvidman, Christian Wejse, and Andreas H. Eiset, "Pregnancy Complications among Refugee Women: A Systematic Review," *Acta Obstetricia et Gynecologica Scandinavica* 100, no. 4 (2021): 649–57.

102. Heather Adair-Rohani, Karen Zukor, Sophie Bonjour, Susan Wilburn, Annette C. Kuesel, Ryan Hebert, and Elaine R. Fletcher, "Limited Electricity Access in Health Facilities of Sub-Saharan Africa: A Systematic Review of Data on Electricity Access, Sources, And Reliability," *Global Health: Science and Practice* 1, no. 2 (2013): 249–61.

103. Edna Kwamboka Moturi, "Appropriate Infection Control Practices in Refugee Camps and Post-conflict Settings" (PhD diss., Emory University, 2011).

104. Gladys Honein-AbouHaidar, Aya Noubani, Nour El Arnaout, Sharif Ismail, Hana Nimer, Marilyne Menassa, Adam P. Coutts, Diana Rayes et al., "Informal Healthcare Provision in Lebanon: An Adaptive Mechanism among Displaced Syrian Health Professionals in a Protracted Crisis," *Conflict and Health* 13, no. 1 (2019): 1–11.

105. Ebiowei S. F. Orubu, Najwa Al-Dheeb, Carly Ching, Sima Bu Jawdeh, Jessica Anderson, Rashad Sheikh, Fadhel Hariri, Huda Basaleem, and Muhammad H. Zaman, "Assessing Antimicrobial Resistance, Utilization and Stewardship in Yemen: An Exploratory Mixed-Methods Study," *American Journal of Tropical Medicine and Hygiene* 105, no. 5 (2021): 1404–12.

106. Jeremy C. Kane, Peter Ventevogel, Paul Spiegel, Judith K. Bass, Mark Van Ommeren, and Wietse A. Tol, "Mental, Neurological, and Substance Use Problems among Refugees in Primary Health Care: Analysis of the Health Information System in 90 Refugee Camps," *BMC Medicine* 12, no. 1 (2014): 1–11.

107. Philippa Boulle, Sylvia Kehlenbrink, James Smith, David Beran, and Kiran Jobanputra, "Challenges Associated with Providing Diabetes Care in Humanitarian Settings," *Lancet Diabetes & Endocrinology* 7, no. 8 (2019): 648–56.

108. Paul Spiegel, Adam Khalifa, and Farrah J. Mateen, "Cancer in Refugees in Jordan and Syria between 2009 and 2012: Challenges and the Way Forward in Humanitarian Emergencies," *Lancet Oncology* 15, no. 7 (2014): e290–e297.

109. Richard A. Powell, Lisa Schwartz, Elysée Nouvet, Brett Sutton, Mila Petrova, Joan Marston, Daniel Munday, and Lukas Radbruch, "Palliative Care in Humanitarian Crises: Always Something to Offer," *Lancet* 389, no. 10078 (2017): 1498–99, https://www.thelancet.com/journals/lancet/article/PIIS0140-6736(17)30978-9/fulltext.

110. Shuait Nair, Aurelia Attal-Juncqua, Aashna Reddy, Erin M. Sorrell, and Claire J. Standley, "Assessing Barriers, Opportunities and Future Directions in Health Information Sharing in Humanitarian Contexts: A Mixed-Method Study," *BMJ Open* 12, no. 4 (2022): e053042.

111. "Lack of Quality Data Compounds Risks Facing Millions of Refugee and Migrant Children," UNICEF, March 2, 2020, https://blogs.unicef.org/evidence-for-action/lack-of-quality-data-compounds-risks-facing-millions-of-displaced-and-migrant-children/.

112. Siyana Mahroof-Shaffi and Bruce Murray, "Data Management Systems for Migrant and Refugee Children," in *Child Refugee and Migrant Health*, ed. Christian Harkensee, Karen Olness, and B. Emily Esmaili (Springer Cham, 2021), 251–66.
113. Sean Wong and Wendy Wang, "Mobile Health Technologies and Medical Records," *University of Western Ontario Medical Journal* 88, no. 1 (2019): 49–51.
114. Russell Hardin, ed., *Distrust* (Russell Sage Foundation, 2004); in particular, chapters by Russell Hardin, Roderick Kramer, and Deborah Larson.
115. Barry Munslow, "Humanitarianism Under Attack," *International Health* 11, no. 5 (2019): 358–60.
116. "More Than 4000 Attacks against Health Workers, Facilities, and Transports since 2016 Underscore Need for Action to Protect Health Care in Conflict," Physicians for Human Rights, May 5, 2021, https://phr.org/news/more-than-4000-attacks-against-health-workers-facilities-and-transports-since-2016-underscore-need-for-action-to-protect-health-care-in-conflict/.
117. "No True Accountability Three Years after Bombing of MSF-supported Hospital," Médecins Sans Frontières press release, October 30, 2019, https://www.msf.org/yemen-hospital-bombing-investigation-findings-too-little-too-late.
118. "When Medical Care Comes under Attack," Médecins Sans Frontières report, 2017(?), https://www.msf.org/attacks-medical-care-depth,
119. For a detailed analysis, see: Leonard Rubenstein, *Perilous Medicine: The Struggle to Protect Health Care from the Violence of War* (Columbia University Press, 2021).
120. Muhammad Hamza Yousuf, Abdul Jabbar, Irfan Ullah, Muhammad Junaid Tahir, and Zohaib Yousaf, "Violence against Health Care System in Areas of Conflict: Unveiling the Crisis Globally," *Ethics, Medicine, and Public Health* 19 (2021): 100730.
121. "Hospitals in Yemen Attacked, Disrupting Healthcare for Thousands of Vulnerable Civilians," UN News (website), February 10, 2020, https://news.un.org/en/story/2020/02/1057101.
122. Rohini J. Haar, Róisín Read, Larissa Fast, Karl Blanchet, Stephanie Rinaldi, Bertrand Taithe, Christina Wille, and Leonard S. Rubenstein, "Violence against Healthcare in Conflict: A Systematic Review of the Literature and Agenda for Future Research," *Conflict and Health* 15, no. 1 (2021): 1–18.

123. Paul B. Spiegel, Francesco Checchi, Sandro Colombo, and Eugene Paik, "Health-Care Needs of People Affected by Conflict: Future Trends and Changing Frameworks," *Lancet* 375, no. 9711 (2010): 341–45.

124. "Violence and Sense of Impunity Force Stop to Lifesaving Care," Médecins Sans Frontières press release, March 21, 2022, https://www.msf.org/violence-and-sense-impunity-halts-lifesaving-care-northeastern-drc.

125. Lindsey N. Kingston, Elizabeth F. Cohen, and Christopher P. Morley, "Debate: Limitations on Universality: The 'Right to Health' and the Necessity of Legal Nationality," *BMC International Health and Human Rights* 10, no. 1 (2010): 1–12.

126. Nefti-Eboni Bempong, Danny Sheath, Joachim Seybold, Antoine Flahault, Anneliese Depoux, and Luciano Saso, "Critical Reflections, Challenges and Solutions for Migrant and Refugee Health: 2nd M8 Alliance Expert Meeting," *Public Health Reviews* 40, no. 1 (2019): 1–12.

127. Adeyinka Abideen Aderinto, "Life after Displacement: A Study of Refugees in a Nigerian Refugee Camp," *Journal of Human Ecology* 13, no. 5 (2002): 369–74.

128. Dene-Hern Chen, "In Rohingya Camps, Traditional Healers Fill a Gap in Helping Refugees Overcome Trauma," *The New Humanitarian*, July 30, 2018, https://www.thenewhumanitarian.org/feature/2018/07/30/rohingya-camps-traditional-healers-fill-gap-helping-refugees-overcome-trauma.

129. Hani Fares and Jaume Puig-Junoy, "Inequity and Benefit Incidence Analysis in Healthcare Use among Syrian Refugees in Egypt," *Conflict and Health* 15, no. 1 (2021): 1–14.

130. Sarah E. Parkinson and Orkideh Behrouzan, "Negotiating Health and Life: Syrian Refugees and the Politics of Access in Lebanon," *Social Science & Medicine* 146 (2015): 324–31.

131. "UNHCR Policy on Refugee Protection and Solutions in Urban Areas," UNHCR, 2009, https://www.unhcr.org/4ab356ab6.pdf.

132. Shannon Doocy, Kathleen R. Page, Fernando De la Hoz, Paul Spiegel, and Chris Beyrer, "Venezuelan Migration and the Border Health Crisis in Colombia and Brazil," *Journal on Migration and Human Security* 7, no. 3 (2019): 79–91.

133. Anastasia Moloney, "As Venezuela's Health System Crumbles, Pregnant Women Flee to Colombia," *Reuters*, June 18, 2018, https://www.reuters

.com/article/colombia-migrants-health/feature-as-venezuelas-health
-system-crumbles-pregnant-women-flee-to-colombia-idUSL5N1T34JJ.

134. "Venezuelans in Colombia Struggle to Find Health Care: 'This Is a
Crisis,'" Relief Web, July 16, 2019, https://reliefweb.int/report/colombia
/venezuelans-colombia-struggle-find-health-care-crisis.

135. "Access to Health Services for Venezuelans in Colombia and Peru
during the COVID-19 Pandemic," Mixed Migration Centre report,
Latin America and the Caribbean 4Mi Snapshot, March 2021, https://
mixedmigration.org/wp-content/uploads/2021/04/167_access_health
_services_Venezuelans_in_Colombia_and_Peru_during_COVID19
.pdf.

136. Joe Parkin Daniels, "Colombia Struggles to Cope with Care in Venezuelan Influx," *Lancet* 393, no. 10187 (2019): 2185–86.

137. Venezuelan Refugees and Migrants in Colombia—Situational Report #4,"
Relief Web, December 31, 2018, https://reliefweb.int/report/colombia
/venezuelan-refugees-and-migrants-colombia-situational-report-4
-december-2018.

138. Sergio Guzmán and Juan Camilo Ponce, "Hate against Venezuelans in
Colombia Is a Ticking Time Bomb," Global Americans (website),
November 10, 2020, https://theglobalamericans.org/2020/11/hate
-against-venezuelans-in-colombia-is-a-ticking-time-bomb/.

139. Julia G. Young, "Making America 1920 Again? Nativism and US Immigration, Past and Present," *Journal on Migration and Human Security* 5, no. 1
(2017): 217–35.

140. "COVID-19 Brief: Impact on Conflict and Refugees," US Global
Leadership Coalition report, April 2022, https://www.usglc.org
/coronavirus/conflict-and-refugees/.

141. Jhinuk Mukhopadhyay and Gauri Thampi, "Persistent COVID-19 Vaccine
Inequity Has Significant Implications for Refugees and Other Vulnerable
Migrants," Migration Policy Institute, April 19, 2022, https://www
.migrationpolicy.org/article/refugees-access-covid-19-vaccine-inequity.

142. "Refugees Receive COVID-19 Vaccinations in Jordan," UNHCR press
release, January 14, 2021, https://www.unhcr.org/en-us/news/press/2021
/1/5fffe614/refugees-receive-covid-19-vaccinations-jordan.html.

143. "Refugees Excluded from COVID-19 Vaccine Rollout according to
World Vision Report," World Vision press release, June 15, 2021, https://

www.worldvision.org/about-us/media-center/refugees-excluded-from
-covid-19-vaccine-rollout-according-to-world-vision-report.

144. Aamir Saeed, "For Pakistan's over Three Million Stateless People,
COVID-19 Jabs Out of Reach," *Arab News*, May 25, 2021, https://www
.arabnews.pk/node/1864586/pakistan.

145. Muhammad Hamid Zaman, Tahera Hasan, and Janki Bhatt, "Invisible
People, Visible Barriers: Healthcare Access for and among Ethnic
Bengalis in Pakistan," *Statelessness & Citizenship Review* 4, no. 2 (2022):
286–92, https://statelessnessandcitizenshipreview.com/index.php
/journal/article/view/357.

146. Samy Magdy, "In Yemen's North, Houthis Face Virus with Outright
Denial," *AP News*, August 12, 2021, https://apnews.com/article/middle
-east-health-coronavirus-pandemic-united-nations-yemen-1d134157c61c8
5c844667613183ac1b3.

147. "Lethal Combination of Climate, Conflict and Covid Sees Humanitarian
Needs Rise by 17% in 2022," ReliefWeb, December 3, 2021, https://
reliefweb.int/report/afghanistan/lethal-combination-climate-conflict
-and-covid-sees-humanitarian-needs-rise-17.

148. Camille Le Coz and Kathleen Newland, "Rewiring Migrant Returns and
Reintegration after the COVID-19 Shock," Migration Policy Institute,
2021, https://reliefweb.int/report/world/rewiring-migrant-returns-and
-reintegration-after-covid-19-shock.

149. "COVID-19 and Afghan Refugees: No Good Options," Refugees
International (website), May 28, 2020, https://www.refugeesinternational
.org/reports/2020/5/28/covid-19-and-afghan-refugees-no-good-options.

150. "Uganda Suspends Refugee Arrivals as Coronavirus Cases Rise," *The New
Humanitarian*, March 25, 2020, https://www.thenewhumanitarian.org
/news/2020/03/25/uganda-coronavirus-refugees-asylum-seekers.

151. Chloe Sydney, "Is It Safe to Return Home? New Research Unpicks
Repeated Displacement in South Sudan," Internal Displacement
Monitoring Centre, November 2019, https://www.internal-displacement
.org/expert-opinion/is-it-safe-to-return-home-new-research-unpicks
-repeated-displacement-in-south-sudan.

152. "Access to Health Care in South Sudan: A Qualitative Analysis of Health
Pooled Fund Supported Counties," Health Pooled Fund, South Sudan,
December 2020, https://www.kit.nl/wp-content/uploads/2021/09
/HPF3-Access-to-healthcare-study-A-qualitative-analysis-report.pdf.

153. Tayseer AlKarim, Lia Harris, and Abdullah Chahin, "WHO Needs Reform: Why and How Syria Was Elected to the WHO Executive Board?," *BMJ Global Health* 6, no. 8 (2021): e006801.

154. Nyagoah Tut Pur, "Surge in Attacks on Aid Workers in South Sudan," Human Rights Watch (website), March 4, 2022, https://www.hrw.org /news/2022/03/04/surge-attacks-aid-workers-south-sudan.

155. "South Sudan Regional Refugee Response Plan, January– December 2022," ReliefWeb, March 17, 2022, https://reliefweb.int /report/uganda/south-sudan-regional-refugee-response-plan-january -december-2022.

156. David Zucchino and Safiullah Padshah, "Afghanistan's Health Care System Is Collapsing Under Stress," *New York Times*, February 14, 2022, https://www.nytimes.com/2022/02/06/world/asia/afghanistans-health -care-system.html.

157. Masood Farivar, "Few Afghan Refugees Relocating to US Under 'P-2' Program," Voice of America, January 12, 2022, https://www.voanews.com/a /few-afghan-refugees-relocating-to-us-under-p-2-program/6394377.html.

158. Philip Whiteside, Kieran Devine, Philip Whiteside, and Johnathan Tooley, "Barbed Wired Borders and the Desert of Death," Sky News (website), https://news.sky.com/story/afghanistan-barbed-wire-borders -and-the-desert-of-death-the-dangerous-escape-routes-facing-refugees -fleeing-the-taliban-12398215.

159. Ali Furqan, "Pakistan Refuses to Host Additional Afghan Refugees," Voice of America, July 13, 2021, https://www.voanews.com/a/south-central-asia _pakistan-refuses-host-additional-afghan-refugees/6208191.html.

160. Ruby Mellen and Júlia Ledur, "Afghanistan Faces Widespread Hunger amid Worsening Humanitarian Crisis," *Washington Post*, January 24, 2022, https://www.washingtonpost.com/world/2022/01/24/afghanistan -humanitarian-crisis-hunger/.

161. Paul Spiegel, "Hospitals Are Collapsing in Afghanistan: At This Rate Sanctions Will Kill More People than the Taliban," *Washington Post*, December 16, 2021, https://www.washingtonpost.com/opinions/2021/12 /16/hospitals-are-collapsing-afghanistan-this-rate-sanctions-will-kill -more-people-than-taliban/.

162. "Pakistan Calls on Muslim Countries to Help Afghanistan," NBC News, December 18, 2021, https://www.nbcnews.com/news/world/pakistan -calls-muslim-countries-help-afghanistan-rcna8870.

163. Shruti Menon, "Afghanistan Earthquake: What Foreign Aid Is Getting In?," BBC News, July 8, 2022, https://www.bbc.com/news/world-asia-59518628.

164. "Taliban Bans Female NGO Staff, Jeopardizing Aid Efforts," *Reuters*, December 24, 2022, https://www.reuters.com/world/asia-pacific/taliban -orders-ngos-ban-female-employees-coming-work-2022-12-24/.

Chapter 4
Trusted Social Networks Help Navigate the System

1. Steven Grattan, "Four Years after FARC Peace Deal, Colombia Grapples with Violence," *Al Jazeera*, November 24, 2020, https://www.aljazeera .com/features/2020/11/24/four-years-after-peace-deal-colombia-grapples -with-violence.

2. Julie Turkewitz, "Colombia Makes 'Historic' Decision to Grant Legal Status to 1.7 Million Venezuelan Migrants," *New York Times*, February 8, 2021, https://www.nytimes.com/2021/02/08/world/americas/colombia -venezuela-migrants-duque.html

3. "Displaced Venezuelans in Colombia Harder Hit By COVID-19 Economic Fallout, New Research Finds," Center for Global Development press release, October 28, 2020, https://www.cgdev.org/article/displaced-venezuelans -colombia-harder-hit-covid-19-economic-fallout-new-research-finds.

4. David Hill, Ellithia Adams, Zafiro Andrade-Romo, Karla Solari, Alfonso Silva Santisteban, and Amaya Perez-Brumer, "Access to COVID-19 Vaccination for Displaced Venezuelans in Latin America: A Rapid Scoping Review," *Lancet Global Health* 10 (2022): S19.

5. "UNHCR Welcomes Colombia's Decision to Regularize Stay of Venezuelans in the Country," UNHCR news briefing, February 4, 2020, https://www.unhcr.org/en-us/news/briefing/2020/2/5e3930db4/unhcr -welcomes-colombias-decision-regularize-stay-venezuelans-country.html.

6. "Episcopal Relief & Development Responds to Civil Unrest and the COVID-19 Pandemic in South Sudan," Relief Web website, April 28, 2022, https://reliefweb.int/report/south-sudan/episcopal-relief -development-responds-civil-unrest-and-covid-19-pandemic-south.

7. Chidochashe L. Munangagwa, "The Economic Decline of Zimbabwe," *Gettysburg Economic Review* 3, no. 1 (2009): 9.

8. Tatenda Chitagu and Rick Noack, "Before Robert Mugabe was hated, he was loved," *Washington Post*, September 6, 2019, https://www.washingtonpost .com/world/2019/09/06/before-robert-mugabe-was-hated-he-was-loved/.

9. For the issue of CNIC and Bengali stateless persons, see Muhammad Hamid Zaman, Tahera Hasan, and Janki Bhatt, "Invisible People, Visible Barriers: Healthcare Access for and among Ethnic Bengalis in Pakistan," *Statelessness & Citizenship Review* 4, no. 2 (2022): 286–92, https://statele ssnessandcitizenshipreview.com/index.php/journal/article/view/357.

10. Tonderayi Mukeredzi, "Power Cuts Are Plaguing Southern Africa: The Region Needs Renewable Energy," *Foreign Policy*, December 24, 2019, https://foreignpolicy.com/2019/12/24/power-cuts-are-plaguing -southern-africa-the-region-needs-renewable-energy/.

11. Kitsepile Nyathi, "Confusion Marks Zimbabwe's Return to Own Currency," *The East African*, June 26, 2019, https://www.theeastafrican.co .ke/tea/news/rest-of-africa/confusion-marks-zimbabwe-s-return-to-own -currency-1421058.

12. Chris Muronzi, "Conceal the Burn: Zimbabwe Is Withholding Official Inflation Data," *Al Jazeera*, August 2, 2019, https://www.aljazeera.com /economy/2019/8/2/conceal-the-burn-zimbabwe-is-withholding-official -inflation-data.

13. Columbus Mavhunga, "Zimbabwe's Economic Crisis Drives Medicine to the Black Market," *Global Citizen*, October 24, 2018, https://www .globalcitizen.org/es/content/zimbabwe-black-market-drugs/.

14. Norimitsu Onishi and Jeffrey Moyo, "Robert Mugabe Resigns as Zimbabwe's President, Ending 37-Year Rule," *New York Times*, November 21, 2017, https://www.nytimes.com/2017/11/21/world/africa /zimbabwe-mugabe-mnangagwa.html.

15. Andrew Mambondiyani, "Zimbabweans Can Hardly Believe This But They Regret Replacing Mugabe with Brutal New Leader," *Daily Beast*, November 30, 2020, https://www.thedailybeast.com/emmerson -mnangagwa-is-even-worse-than-robert-mugabe-zimbabwe-regrets-coup.

16. Godfrey Chikowore, "Contradictions in Development Aid: The Case of Zimbabwe," in *South-South Cooperation: A Challenge to the Aid System?*, The Reality of Aid Network Special Report on South-South Cooperation, 2010, 45.

17. Jeffrey Moyo, "Renewed Exodus of Zimbabweans amid Economic Woes," Anadolu Agency, October 27, 2019, https://www.aa.com.tr/en/africa /renewed-exodus-of-zimbabweans-amid-economic-woes/1627663.

18. Jonathan Crush, Godfrey Tawodzera, Abel Chikanda, Sujata Ramachandran, and Daniel Tevera, "South Africa Case Study: The Double

Crisis—Mass Migration from Zimbabwe and Xenophobic Violence in
South Africa," Migrants in Countries in Crisis, International Centre for
Migration Policy Development, January 2017.

19. Fainos Mangena, "Hunhu/Ubuntu in the Traditional Thought of
Southern Africa," Internet Encyclopedia of Philosophy (website), 2016.

20. Vicky Cattell, "Poor People, Poor Places, and Poor Health: The Mediat-
ing Role of Social Networks and Social Capital," *Social Science &
Medicine* 52, no. 10 (2001): 1501–16.

21. Kirsten P. Smith and Nicholas A. Christakis, "Social Networks and
Health," *Annual Review of Sociology* 34, no. 1 (2008): 405–29.

22. Jaber Suleiman, "Marginalised Community: The Case of Palestinian
Refugees in Lebanon," Development Research Centre on Migration,
Globalisation and Poverty, 2006, 12.

23. Manal Kortam, "Politics, Patronage and Popular Committees in the
Shatila Refugee Camp, Lebanon," in *Palestinian Refugees*, ed. Are
Knudsen and Sari Hanafi (Routledge, 2010), 207–18.

24. For UNRWA camp in Shatila, see "Shatila Camp," https://www.unrwa
.org/where-we-work/lebanon/shatila-camp.

25. S. Khoury, T. Graczyk, G. Burnham, M. Jurdi, and L. Goldman, "Drinking Water System Treatment and Contamination in Shatila Refugee
Camp in Beirut, Lebanon," *Eastern Mediterranean Health Journal* 22,
no. 8 (2016): 568–78.

26. Dani Abi Ghanem, "Infrastructure and the Vulnerability of Palestinian
Refugees in Lebanon: The Story of Shatila Camp's 'Electricity Matyrs,'"
Jadaliyya, January 2, 2020, https://www.jadaliyya.com/Details/40397.

27. Leila Shahid, "The Sabra and Shatila Massacres: Eye-witness Reports,"
Journal of Palestine Studies 32, no. 1 (2002): 36–58.

28. Maja Janmyr, "Precarity in Exile: The Legal Status of Syrian Refugees in
Lebanon," *Refugee Survey Quarterly* 35, no. 4 (2016): 58–78.

29. Nell Gabiam, *The Politics of Suffering: Syria's Palestinian Refugee Camps*
(Indiana University Press, 2016).

30. Birgitte Stampe Holst, "On the Inside: Shatila Camp as a Space of
Respite for Syrian Refugees," *Journal of Refugee Studies* 35, no. 3 (2022):
1311–26.

31. Lars Erslev Andersen, "The Neglected: Palestinian Refugees in Lebanon
and the Syrian Refugee Crisis," Danish Institute for International Studies
Report, No. 2016: 12 (2016).

32. Omer Karasapan and Sajjad Shah, "Why Syrian Refugees in Lebanon Are a Crisis within a Crisis," Brookings Institution (website), April 15, 2021.

33. Anchal Vohra, "Syrian Refugees' Plight in Lebanon 10 Years after the Uprising," *Al Jazeera*, March 19, 2021, https://www.aljazeera.com/news /2021/3/19/syrian-refugees-in-lebanon-ten-years-after-the-uprising.

34. Jessy Nassar and Nora Stel, "Lebanon's Response to the Syrian Refugee Crisis: Institutional Ambiguity as a Governance Strategy," *Political Geography* 70 (2019): 44–54.

35. Hanadi Syam, Emilie Venables, Bernard Sousse, Nathalie Severy, Luz Saavedra, and Francois Kazour, "'With Every Passing Day I Feel Like a Candle, Melting Little by Little': Experiences of Long-term Displacement amongst Syrian Refugees in Shatila, Lebanon," *Conflict and Health* 13, no. 1 (2019): 1–12.

36. Personal communication of the author with UNHCR and UNRWA Staff. See also: Flora Haderer, Emilie Venables, Josefien van Olmen, Miriam Orcutt, Michella Ghassibe-Sabbagh, and Wilma van den Boogaard, "'I Try the One That They Say Is Good': Factors Influencing Choice of Health Care Provider and Pathways to Diabetes Care for Syrian Refugees in Lebanon," *Conflict and Health* 15, no. 1 (2021): 1–11.

37. "Syrian Refugees in Lebanon Desperate for Health Care amid International Apathy," Amnesty International press release, May 2014, https:// www.amnesty.org/en/latest/news/2014/05/syrian-refugees-lebanon -desperate-health-care-amid-international-apathy/.

38. Personal communication of the author with UNHCR and UNRWA Staff.

39. Jennifer Ibrahim, "The Discrimination against Palestinian Refugees Living in Lebanon," *Palestine-Israel Journal of Politics, Economics, and Culture* 15, no. 1–2 (2008): 83.

40. Marjolein Winters, Bernd Rechel, Lea De Jong, and Milena Pavlova, "A Systematic Review on the Use of Healthcare Services by Undocumented Migrants in Europe," *BMC Health Services Research* 18, no. 1 (2018): 1–10.

41. Winters et al., "Systematic Review."

42. Dipanjan Roy Chaudhury, "Bengali-speaking Muslims Languish in Pakistan," *Economic Times*, October 28, 2019, https://economictimes .indiatimes.com/news/international/world-news/bengali-speaking -muslims-languish-in-pakistan/articleshow/71792488.cms.

43. Personal communication of the author with staff of Imkaan Welfare in Karachi.

44. Marieke Wissink and Valentina Mazzucato, "In Transit: Changing Social Networks of Sub-Saharan African Migrants in Turkey and Greece," *Social Networks* 53 (2018): 30–41.

45. Maude Ulrika, "Local Social Networks Often Involve Ties with other Migrants: A Case of Integration Process," *European Journal of Migration, Diaspora and Remittances* 18, no 6 (2018), https://papers.ssrn.com/sol3 /papers.cfm?abstract_id=3809117.

46. Markus Balázs Göransson, Lotta Hultin, and Magnus Mähring, "'The Phone Means Everything': Mobile Phones, Livelihoods and Social Capital among Syrian Refugees in Informal Tented Settlements in Lebanon," *Migration and Development* 9, no. 3 (2020): 331–51.

47. Bram Frouws, Melissa Phillips, Ashraf Hassan, and Mirjam Twigt, "Getting to Europe the WhatsApp Way: The Use of ICT in Contemporary Mixed Migration Flows to Europe," Regional Mixed Migration Secretariat briefing paper, June 2016.

48. Marie Gillespie, Lawrence Ampofo, Margaret Cheesman, Becky Faith, Evgenia Iliadou, Ali Issa, Souad Osseiran, and Dimitris Skleparis, "Mapping Refugee Media Journeys: Smartphones and Social Media Networks," The Open University, May 13, 2016, https://eprints.ncl.ac .uk/file_store/production/259734/B10ABC43-B969-41E5-A53B -AB553958E6F8.pdf.

49. Helen Mackreath, "The Role of Host Communities in North Lebanon," *Forced Migration Review* 47 (2014): 19,

50. Margaret Kay, Shanika Wijayanayaka, Harriet Cook, and Samantha Hollingworth, "Understanding Quality Use of Medicines in Refugee Communities in Australian Primary Care: A Qualitative Study," *British Journal of General Practice* 66, no. 647 (2016): e397-e409.

51. Rianne Dekker, Godfried Engbersen, Jeanine Klaver, and Hanna Vonk, "Smart Refugees: How Syrian Asylum Migrants Use Social Media Information in Migration Decision-making," *Social Media + Society* 4, no. 1 (2018): 2056305118764439.

52. Kevin Pottie, Ayesha Ratnayake, Rukhsana Ahmed, Luisa Veronis, and Idris Alghazali, "How Refugee Youth Use Social Media: What Does This Mean for Improving Their Health and Welfare?," *Journal of Public Health Policy* 41, no. 3 (2020): 268–78.

53. Katharine M. Donato, Lisa Singh, Ali Arab, Elizabeth Jacobs, and Douglas Post, "Misinformation about COVID-19 and Venezuelan

Migration: Trends in Twitter Conversation during a Pandemic," *Harvard Data Science Review* 4, no. 1 (2022).

54. Tiziana Mancini, Federica Sibilla, Dimitris Argiropoulos, Michele Rossi, and Marina Everri, "The Opportunities and Risks of Mobile Phones for Refugees' Experience: A Scoping Review," *PLOS One* 14, no. 12 (2019): e0225684.

55. Shira Rubin, "Desperate Refugees Sell Their Own Organs To Survive," Vocativ (website), February 24, 2017, https://www.vocativ.com/404068 /desperate-refugees-organs-black-market/index.html.

Chapter 5
Unregulated Medical Practices and Providers

1. Matthew Bristow and Marie Monteleone, "Vital Food and Fuel Exit Venezuela as Smuggling Worsens Crisis," *Bloomberg News*, February 19, 2019, https://www.bloomberg.com/news/photo-essays/2019-02-19/vital -food-and-fuel-exit-venezuela-as-smuggling-worsens-crisis.

2. James Bargent, "Cucuta: Colombia's Contraband City," InSight Crime, November 16, 2014, https://insightcrime.org/news/analysis/cucuta -colombia-contraband-city/.

3. Ezra Kaplan, "Inside the Booming Smuggling Trade Between Venezuela and Colombia," *TIME*, March 31, 2016, https://time.com/4254619/inside -the-booming-smuggling-trade-between-venezuela-and-colombia/.

4. Laura Jayne Dixon, "Heading Far Afield to Enter Motherhood," *US News*, November 27, 2019, https://www.usnews.com/news/best-countries/articles /2019-11-27/pregnant-venezuelan-women-flood-colombias-hospitals.

5. Anggy Polanco and Isaac Urrutia, "Venezuela's Chronic Shortages Give Rise to 'Medical Flea Markets,'" *Reuters*, December 8, 2017, https://www .reuters.com/article/us-venezuela-medicine/venezuelas-chronic-shortages -give-rise-to-medical-flea-markets-idUSKBN1E21J4.

6. "Venezuelans Smuggling Medicine, Food across Colombia Border in order to Feed Themselves, Families," Global News Canada, February 20, 2019, https://globalnews.ca/video/4979479/venezuelans-smuggling -medicine-food-across-colombia-border-in-order-to-feed-themselves -families.

7. Juan Diego Cárdenas, "Coronavirus Stokes Colombia's Black Market Medicine Trade," InSight Crime (website), April 16, 2020, https:// insightcrime.org/news/brief/coronavirus-colombia-medicine/.

8. Johanna Aponte-González, Angélica González-Acuña, José Lopez, Paul Brown, and Javier Eslava-Schmalbach, "Perceptions in the Community about the Use of Antibiotics without a Prescription: Exploring Ideas behind this Practice," *Pharmacy Practice* (Granada) 17, no. 1 (2019).

9. Patricio Zambrano-Barragán, Sebastián Ramírez Hernández, Luisa Feline Freier, Marta Luzes, Rita Sobczyk, Alexander Rodríguez, and Charles Beach, "The Impact of COVID-19 on Venezuelan Migrants' Access to Health: A Qualitative Study in Colombian and Peruvian Cities," *Journal of Migration and Health* 3 (2021): 100029.

10. Anastasia Moloney, "In Colombia, Abortion Is Legal but Denied to Many Women, Advocates Say," *Reuters*, May 25, 2016, https://www.reuters.com/article/us-abortion-colombia-law/in-colombia-abortion-is-legal-but-denied-to-many-women-advocates-say-idUSKCN0YG1GX.

11. Anastasia Moloney, "Venezuela Crisis Forces Women to Sell Sex in Colombia, Fuels Slavery Risk," *Reuters Japan*, June 5, 2017, https://jp.reuters.com/article/us-venezuela-colombia-trafficking-idUSKBN18W1EX.

12. Khabir Ahmad, "Herbal Treatment for HIV/AIDS Not Recommended," *Lancet Infectious Diseases* 5, no. 9 (2005): 537.

13. Médecins Sans Frontières, "International Activity Report: Pakistan," 2017, https://www.msf.org/international-activity-report-2017/pakistan.

14. Farhan Mushtaq, "Faith Healing: An Unregulated Health Domain" (graduate research project, Institute of Business Administration, Pakistan, 2019), https://ir.iba.edu.pk/research-projects-msj/13/.

15. There are frequent reports in local newspapers about abuse. For example, a search of the terms *abuse + faith healers + Pakistan* leads to hundreds of stories and articles over several years. See, for example: Alex Rodriguez, "In Pakistan, Faith Healers Have No Shortage of Believers," *Los Angeles Times*, March 29, 2012, https://www.latimes.com/world/la-xpm-2012-mar-29-la-fg-pakistan-superstition-20120330-story.html. Also see: Alizeh Kohari, "Jinnfluencers: Inside the World of Internet Exorcisms," *The Juggernaut*, February 9, 2021, https://www.thejuggernaut.com/jinnfluencers-inside-the-world-of-internet-exorcisms.

16. Noman Ahmed, "The Talking Walls of Karachi," *Dawn*, January 9, 2022, https://www.dawn.com/news/1668478; also available at Urban Resource Centre Karachi (website), https://urckarachi.org/2022/01/31/the-talking-walls-of-karachi.

17. Alvin Kuowei Tay, Andrew Riley, Rafiqul Islam, Courtney Welton-Mitchell, Benedicte Duchesne, V. Waters, Andrea Varner, B. Moussa et al., "The Culture, Mental Health and Psychosocial Wellbeing of Rohingya Refugees: A Systematic Review," *Epidemiology and Psychiatric Sciences* 28, no. 5 (2019): 489–94.

18. Sujata Regina Swaroop, "Phenomenological Perspectives on Internal Displacement and Healing: Implications for Evidence-based Therapies" (PhD diss., Chicago School of Professional Psychology, 2013), https://www.proquest.com/docview/1430985637.

19. Swaroop, "Phenomenological Perspectives."

20. Farida Pirani, "Therapeutic Encounters at a Muslim Shrine in Pakistan: An Ethnographic Study of Understandings and Explanations of Ill Health and Help-Seeking among Attenders" (PhD diss., Middlesex University, 2009).

21. "Deaths Due to Tainted Herbal Medicine Under-Recorded," *Science Daily*, October 25, 2018, https://www.sciencedaily.com/releases/2018/10/181025103344.htm.

22. Babar T. Shaikh and Juanita Hatcher, "Complementary and Alternative Medicine in Pakistan: Prospects and Limitations," *Evidence-Based Complementary and Alternative Medicine* 2, no. 2 (2005): 139–42.

23. Asif Mehmood, "How Faith Healers Prey on the Most Vulnerable," *The Express Tribune*, March 5, 2022, https://tribune.com.pk/story/2346428/how-faith-healers-prey-on-the-most-vulnerable.

24. Mohammad Ali, Bilal Haider Abbasi, Nisar Ahmad, Hina Fazal, Jafar Khan, and Syed Shujait Ali, "Over-the-Counter Medicines in Pakistan: Misuse and Overuse," *Lancet* 395, no. 10218 (2020): 116.

25. Mariyam Sarfraz and Saima Hamid, "Challenges in Delivery of Skilled Maternal Care: Experiences of Community Midwives in Pakistan," *BMC Pregnancy and Childbirth* 14, no. 1 (2014): 1–13.

26. Sunaina Kumar, "Why Rohingya Women Risk Dangerous Home Births in Bangladesh's Refugee Camps," *The New Humanitarian*, June 3, 2019, https://www.thenewhumanitarian.org/news/2019/06/03/why-rohingya-women-risk-dangerous-home-births-bangladesh-s-refugee-camps.

27. Andrea Nove, Sally Pairman, Leah F. Bohle, Shantanu Garg, Nester T. Moyo, Michaela Michel-Schuldt, Axel Hoffmann, and Gonçalo Castro, "The Development of a Global Midwifery Education Accreditation Programme," *Global Health Action* 11, no. 1 (2018): 1489604.

28. Filby, Alex, Fran McConville, and Anayda Portela. "What Prevents Quality Midwifery Care? A Systematic Mapping of Barriers in Low and Middle Income Countries from the Provider Perspective," *PLOS One* 11, no. 5 (2016): e0153391.

29. Merveille Kavira Luneghe, "Lacking Access to Medical Childbirth, Pygmies and Displaced Women in DRC Turn to Untrained Midwives," *Global Press Journal*, January 21, 2015, https://globalpressjournal.com /africa/democratic-republic-of-congo/lacking-access-to-medical -childbirth-pygmies-and-displaced-women-in-drc-turn-to-untrained -midwives/.

30. Tensae Mekonnen, Tinashe Dune, Janette Perz, and Felix Akpojene Ogbo, "Trends and Predictors of the Use of Unskilled Birth Attendants among Ethiopian Mothers from 2000 to 2016," *Sexual & Reproductive Healthcare* 28 (2021): 100594.

31. Decio Ribeiro Sarmento, "Traditional Birth Attendance (TBA) in a Health System: What Are the Roles, Benefits and Challenges: A Case Study of Incorporated TBA in Timor-Leste," *Asia Pacific Family Medicine* 13, no. 1 (2014): 1–9.

32. Waqas Hameed and Bilal Iqbal Avan, "Women's Experiences of Mistreatment during Childbirth: A Comparative View of Home- and Facility-based Births in Pakistan," *PLOS One* 13, no. 3 (2018): e0194601.

33. Faith C. Diorgu and Awoala N. George, "Broader Driver of Disrespectful Maternity Care: Power Dynamics," *Obstetrics & Gynecology* 3 (2021): 130–33.

34. Umar Bacha, "Maternal, Newborn Health at Risk in KP's Shangla Due to Unregistered Clinics, Unqualified Medics," Relief Web (website), December 23, 2019, https://reliefweb.int/report/pakistan/maternal -newborn-health-risk-kps-shangla-due-unregistered-clinics-unqualified -medics.

35. Muhammad Asim, Sehrish Karim, Hajra Khwaja, Waqas Hameed, and Sarah Saleem, "The Unspoken Grief of Multiple Stillbirths in Rural Pakistan: An Interpretative Phenomenological Study," *BMC Women's Health* 22, no. 1 (2022): 1–11.

36. Asif Raza Khowaja, Craig Mitton, Rahat Qureshi, Stirling Bryan, Laura A. Magee, Peter von Dadelszen, and Zulfiqar A. Bhutta, "A Comparison of Maternal and Newborn Health Services Costs in Sindh Pakistan," *PLOS One* 13, no. 12 (2018): e0208299.

37. Maksuma Akter, "I Am a Midwife in a Rohingya Refugee Camp—Here's What It's Like," Intrahealth (website), May 7, 2020, https://www.intrahealth .org/vital/i-am-midwife-rohingya-refugee-camp—here's-what-it's.

38. M. Saeed Siddiqui, M. Khalid Siddiqui, and Aijaz Ahmad Sohag, "Health Seeking Behavior of the People: Knowledge, Attitudes and Practices (KAP) Study of the People of Urban Slum Areas of Karachi," *Professional Medical Journal* 18, no. 04 (2011): 626–31.

39. Shershah Syed, "Health: The Lure of Quacks," *Dawn*, November 4, 2018, https://www.dawn.com/news/1443342.

40. Jean Pierre Hiegel, "Use of Indigenous Concepts and Healers in the Care of Refugees: Some Experiences from the Thai Border Camps," in *Amidst Peril and Pain: The Mental Health and Well-Being of the World's Refugees*, ed. A. J. Marsella, T. Bornemann, S. Ekblad, and J. Orley (American Psychological Association, 1994), 293–309.

41. Muhammad Zaid, Muhammad Ali, and Muhammad Sohail Afzal, "HIV Outbreaks in Pakistan," *Lancet HIV* 6, no. 7 (2019): e418-e419.

42. Aimee Lehmann, "Safe Abortion: A Right for Refugees?," *Reproductive Health Matters* 10, no. 19 (2002): 151–55.

43. Camille Pabalan, "Abortion Care in Humanitarian Conflict-Affected Settings: A Scoping Review" (research article, University of Ottawa, 2020).

44. Clémentine Rossier, Angela Marchin, Caron Kim, and Bela Ganatra, "Disclosure to Social Network Members among Abortion-Seeking Women in Low- and Middle-Income Countries with Restrictive Access: A Systematic Review," *Reproductive Health* 18, no. 1 (2021): 1–15.

45. Blake Erhardt-Ohren and Sarah Lewinger, "Refugee and Internally Displaced Women's Abortion Knowledge, Attitudes and Practices: Addressing the Lack of Research in Low- and Middle-Income Countries," *International Perspectives on Sexual and Reproductive Health* 46, Supplement 1 (2020): 77–81.

46. Shalika Hegde, Elizabeth Hoban, and Annemarie Nevill, "Unsafe Abortion as a Birth Control Method: Maternal Mortality Risks among Unmarried Cambodian Migrant Women on the Thai-Cambodia Border," *Asia Pacific Journal of Public Health* 24, no. 6 (2012): 989–1001.

47. "Lebanon Refugee Crisis: Pharmacists Have Huge Potential in the Refugee Crisis But Must Act Now," International Pharmaceutical Federation (website), May 14 2019, https://www.fip.org/lebanon-refugee -crisis.

48. Azhar Hussain and Mohamed Izham M. Ibrahim, "Qualification, Knowledge and Experience of Dispensers Working at Community Pharmacies in Pakistan," *Pharmacy Practice* 9, no. 2 (2011): 93.

49. Saira Azhar, Mohamed Azmi Hassali, Mohamed Izham Mohamed Ibrahim, Maqsood Ahmad, Imran Masood, and Asrul Akmal Shafie, "The Role of Pharmacists in Developing Countries: The Current Scenario in Pakistan," *Human Resources for Health* 7, no. 1 (2009): 1–6.

50. Danielle A. Badro, Hala Sacre, Souheil Hallit, Ali Amhaz, and Pascale Salameh, "Good Pharmacy Practice Assessment among Community Pharmacies in Lebanon," *Pharmacy Practice (Granada)* 18, no. 1 (2020).

51. Chhorvoin Om, Frances Daily, Erika Vlieghe, James C. McLaughlin, and Mary-Louise McLaws, "Pervasive Antibiotic Misuse in the Cambodian Community: Antibiotic-Seeking Behaviour with Unrestricted Access," *Antimicrobial Resistance & Infection Control* 6, no. 1 (2017): 1–8.

52. Majdoleen Al Alawneh, Nabeel Nuaimi, Eman Abu-Gharbieh, and Iman A. Basheti, "A Randomized Control Trial Assessing the Effect of a Pharmaceutical Care Service on Syrian Refugees' Quality of Life and Anxiety," *Pharmacy Practice (Granada)* 18, no. 1 (2020).

53. Report on the 70th World Health Assembly, Pan American Health Organization, May 29, 2017, https://www.paho.org/en/news/29-5-2017-delegates-world-health-assembly-have-reached-new-agreements-dementia-immunization.

54. Justin Dixon, Eleanor MacPherson, and Salome Manyau, "The 'Drug Bag' Method: Antibiotic Stories in Harare, Zimbabwe," Antimicrobials in Society (website), September 25, 2018, https://antimicrobialsinsociety.org/commentary/the-drug-bag-method-antibiotic-stories-in-harare-zimbabwe/.

55. N. Nyazema, N. Viberg, S. Khoza, S. Vyas, L. Kumaranayake, G. Tomson, and C. Stålsby Lundborg, "Low Sale of Antibiotics without Prescription: A Cross-Sectional Study in Zimbabwean Private Pharmacies," *Journal of Antimicrobial Chemotherapy* 59, no. 4 (2007): 718–26.

56. Sifelani Tsiko, "AMR Study Reveals Shocking Misuse of Antibiotics in Zimbabwe," *Zimbabwe Herald*, January 17, 2017, https://www.herald.co.zw/amr-study-reveals-shocking-misuse-of-antibiotics-in-zim/.

57. "Trading in Venezuela's Pain: Border Vendors Do Brisk Business in Meds," France 24 News (website), February 10, 2019, https://www.france24.com/en/20190210-trading-venezuelas-pain-border-vendors-do-brisk-business-meds.

58. Zeina Sahloul, "Challenges Providing Pharmaceutical Products to Syrian Refugees," Regulatory Focus (a publication of Regulatory Affairs Professional Society), May 24, 2017, https://www.raps.org/regulatory -focus%E2%84%A2/news-articles/2017/5/challenges-providing -pharmaceutical-products-to-syrian-refugees.

59. World Health Organization, "Migration and Health: Key Issues," https:// www.euro.who.int/__data/assets/pdf_file/0005/293270/Migration-Health -Key-Issues-.pdf.

60. Muhammad H. Zaman, Biography of Resistance (Harper Collins, 2020).

Chapter 6
Accessing Health Care via Digital Technologies

1. "Homelessness in South Sudan," The Borgen Project (website), https:// borgenproject.org/category/south-sudan/page/4/.

2. Aasim Saleem, "Denial and Conspiracy Theories Fuel Coronavirus Crisis," Deutsche Welle (DW) (website), June 23, 2020, https://www.dw.com/en /how-denial-and-conspiracy-theories-fuel-coronavirus-crisis-in-pakistan/a -53913842.

3. Waqar Gillani, "Dangerous Theories," The News (Pakistan), June 21, 2020, https://www.thenews.com.pk/tns/detail/674847-dangerous-theorie.

4. Jessie Yeung and Sophia Saifi, "Vaccines Sell Out in Pakistan as the Private Market Opens, Raising Concerns of Inequality," CNN (website), April 12, 2021, https://www.cnn.com/2021/04/12/asia/pakistan-covid -private-vaccines-dst-intl-hnk/index.html.

5. "Many Karachiites Fall for Covid Vaccine Myths," Express Tribune, January 14, 2022, https://tribune.com.pk/story/2338664/many -karachiites-fall-for-covid-vaccine-myths.

6. Regarding statelessness and CNIC issues in Pakistan, see for example: Xari Jalil, "50 Years of Statelessness: The Bengalis of Macchar Colony," Voicepk.net, December 27, 2021, https://voicepk.net/2021/12/50-years -of-statelessness-the-bengalis-of-macchar-colony/.

7. Sumaira Jajja, "Citizens without CNICs Eligible for Covid-19 Vaccination in Karachi," Dawn, August 2, 2021, https://www.dawn.com/news /1638388.

8. Sally Hayden, "For Refugees in Detention Camps, Smartphones Are a Lifeline," Wired, March 29, 2022, https://www.wired.com/story/refugees -migration-technology/.

9. Elizabeth Mearns, "Why Smartphones Can Be More Important for Refugees Than Healthcare," CGTN News, October 16, 2019, https:// newseu.cgtn.com/news/2019-09-18/The-digital-divide-in-refugee-camps -JSTsV208Te/index.html.

10. Ivy Kaplan, "How Smartphones and Social Media Have Revolutionized Refugee Migration," UNHCR (blog), October 26, 2018, https://www .unhcr.org/blogs/smartphones-revolutionized-refugee-migration/.

11. Hanna Kozlowska, "The Most Crucial Item That Migrants and Refugees Carry Is a Smartphone," *Quartz*, September 14, 2015, https://qz.com /500062/the-most-crucial-item-that-migrants-and-refugees-carry-is-a -smartphone/.

12. Sveta Milusheva, Daniel Björkegren, and Leonardo Viotti, "Can We Trust Smartphone Mobility Estimates in Low-Income Countries?," World Bank (blog), October 18, 2021, https://blogs.worldbank.org/opendata/can-we -trust-smartphone-mobility-estimates-low-income-countries.

13. Paula Gilbert, "Sub-Saharan Africa Still Struggling with Mobile Gender Gap," Connecting Africa (website), May 3, 2020, https://www .connectingafrica.com/author.asp?section_id=761&doc_id=758009.

14. Anam Feroz, Rawshan Jabeen, and Sarah Saleem, "Using Mobile Phones to Improve Community Health Workers Performance in Low- and Middle-Income Countries," *BMC Public Health* 20, no. 1 (2020): 1–6.

15. Amanda Alencar, Katerina Kondova, and Wannes Ribbens, "The Smartphone as a Lifeline: An Exploration of Refugees' Use of Mobile Communication Technologies during Their Flight," *Media, Culture & Society* 41, no. 6 (2019): 828–44.

16. Olivier Laurent, "The Messages That Hold Refugee Families Together," *TIME Magazine*, March 28, 2016, https://time.com/4272666/refugees -stories-whatsapp/.

17. Karima Manji, Johanna Hanefeld, Jo Vearey, Helen Walls, and Thea de Gruchy, "Using Whatsapp Messenger for Health Systems Research: A Scoping Review of Available Literature," *Health Policy and Planning* 36, no. 5 (2021): 774–89.

18. "Mexico: Migrants Using Whatsapp Can Get Advice on How to Stay Safe and Avoid Illness, Sickness," Relief Web (website), April 3, 2019, https://reliefweb.int/report/mexico/mexico-migrants-using-whatsapp -can-get-advice-how-stay-safe-and-avoid-illness-sickness.

19. "From Digital Promise to Frontline Practice: New and Emerging Technologies in Humanitarian Action," Relief Web (website), April 19, 2021, https://reliefweb.int/report/world/digital-promise-frontline -practice-new-and-emerging-technologies-humanitarian-action.

20. "How Improved Data Could Boost Humanitarian Investment," World Economic Forum (website), March 2, 2021, https://www.weforum.org /agenda/2021/03/improved-data-boost-humanitarian-investment/.

21. Meghan Benton, "Digital Litter: The Downside of Using Technology to Help Refugees," Migration Policy Insitute, June 20, 2019, https://www .migrationpolicy.org/article/digital-litter-downside-using-technology -help-refugees.

22. Bethan Staton, "Eye Spy: Biometric Aid System Trials in Jordan," *The New Humanitarian*, May 18, 2016, https://www.thenewhumanitarian.org /analysis/2016/05/18/eye-spy-biometric-aid-system-trials-jordan.

23. Petra Molnar, "Territorial and Digital Borders and Migrant Vulnerability Under a Pandemic Crisis," In *Migration and Pandemics*, ed. Anna Triandafyllidou, 45–64 (Springer Cham, 2022).

24. Miriam Ganslmeier, "Data Privacy for Migrants: Unrealistic or Simply Neglected?," Heinrich Böll Foundation, October 29, 2019, https://us .boell.org/en/2019/10/29/data-privacy-migrants-unrealistic-or-simply -neglected.

25. Caroline O'Donovan, "Tracking Refugees Puts a Vulnerable Population at Risk," *Buzzfeed News*, December 7, 2015, https://www.buzzfeednews .com/article/carolineodonovan/tracking-refugees-puts-a-vulnerable -population-at-risk.

26. Sneha Indrajit, "The Cybersecurity Risks of Using Biometric Data to Issue Refugee Aid," The Henry M. Jackson School of International Studies (website), July 25 2017, https://jsis.washington.edu/news /cybersecurity-risks-using-biometric-data-issue-refugee-aid/.

27. "UN Shared Rohingya Data without Informed Consent," Human Rights Watch (website), June 15, 2021, https://www.hrw.org/news/2021/06/15 /un-shared-rohingya-data-without-informed-consent.

28. Zara Rahman, "The UN's Refugee Data Shame," The New Humanitarian, June 21, 2021, https://www.thenewhumanitarian.org/opinion/2021 /6/21/rohingya-data-protection-and-UN-betrayal.

29. "UN Shared Rohingya Data."

30. Catriona Mackenzie, Christopher McDowell, and Eileen Pittaway, "Beyond 'Do No Harm': The Challenge of Constructing Ethical Relationships in Refugee Research," *Journal of Refugee Studies* 20, no. 2 (2007): 299–319.

31. Kerrie Holloway, Reem Al Masri, and A. Abu Yahi, *Digital Identity, Biometrics and Inclusion in Humanitarian Responses to Refugee Crises*, Humanitarian Policy Group working paper, ODI, https://cdn.odi.org /media/documents/Digital_IP_Biometrics_case_study_web. pdf.

32. Rahman, "UN's Refugee Data Shame."

33. "Pakistan: Smartcard Registration Drive for Afghan Refugees Ends," *UN News*, January 4, 2022, https://news.un.org/en/story/2022/01/1109062.

34. Eve Hayes de Kalaf, "How Some Countries Are Using Digital ID to Exclude Vulnerable People around the World," The Conversation (website), August 3, 2021, https://theconversation.com/how-some-countries-are -using-digital-id-to-exclude-vulnerable-people-around-the-world-164879.

35. Anadolu Agency, "3 Million People in Pakistan Lacking IDs May Miss Out on COVID-19 Jabs," *Dawn*, May 22, 2021, https://www.dawn.com /news/1625073.

36. Sumaira Jajja, "Citizens without CNICs Eligible for COVID-19 Vaccination in Karachi," *Dawn*, August 2, 2021, https://www.dawn.com/news/1638388.

37. "CNICs of Biharis/Bengalis: Discrimination by Nadra and Nara Criticised," *Business Recorder*, December 16, 2004, https://www.brecorder.com /news/3110905/cnics-of-biharisbengalis-discrimination-by-nadra-and-nara -criticised-2004121688482.

38. "Nadra Alien Registration Card / Nadra Alien Card," My Urdu World (YouTube), August 20, 2021, https://www.youtube.com/watch?v=78F7 _WbiQ2s.

39. de Kalaf, "How Some Countries Are Using Digital ID to Exclude."

40. Molly Bode, Tristan Goodrich, Marilyn Kimeu, Peter Okebukola, and Matt Wilson, "Unlocking Digital Healthcare in Lower- and Middle- Income Countries," McKinsey Report, November 10, 2021, https://www .mckinsey.com/industries/healthcare-systems-and-services/our-insights /unlocking-digital-healthcare-in-lower-and-middle-income-countries.

41. Maeve Shearlaw, "A Cellphone Is No Substitute for a Midwife, African Tech Prodigy Warns," *Guardian*, December 6, 2016, https://www .theguardian.com/world/2016/dec/06/a-cellphone-is-no-substitute-for -a-midwife-african-tech-prodigy-warns.

42. Sy Atezaz Saeed and Ross MacRae Masters, "Disparities in Health Care and the Digital Divide," *Current Psychiatry Reports* 23, no. 9 (2021): 1–6.

43. Devika Nadkarni, Imad Elhajj, Zaher Dawy, Hala Ghattas, and Muhammad H. Zaman, "Examining the Need and Potential for Biomedical Engineering to Strengthen Health Care Delivery for Displaced Populations and Victims of Conflict," *Conflict and Health* 11, no. 1 (2017): 1–4.

44. Nadkarni et al., "Examining the Need and Potential for Biomedical Engineering."

45. For more on Humanitarian Grand Challenges, see https://humanitariangrandchallenge.org/innovator/mobility-for-all/.

46. Conner Evans, Andrew Parsons, Madiha Samadi, Jamie Seah, and Caroline Wallace, "Leveraging Humanitarian Technology to Assist Refugees," Perry World House, University of Pennsylvania, 2017, https://global.upenn.edu/sites/default/files/perry-world-house/Humanitarian TechnologyReport1.pdf.

47. Shelly Culbertson, James Dimarogonas, Katherine Costello, and Serafina Lanna, *Crossing the Digital Divide: Applying Technology to the Global Refugee Crisis* (RAND Corporation, 2019).

48. Nadkarni et al., "Examining the Need and Potential for Biomedical Engineering."

49. Paul B. Spiegel, "The Humanitarian System Is Not Just Broke, But Broken: Recommendations for Future Humanitarian Action," *Lancet* (2017): S0140-6736(17)31278-3.

50. International Federation of Red Cross and Red Crescent Societies, "NCD [Noncommunicable Disease] Care in Humanitarian Settings: A Clarion Call to Civil Society," 2021, https://www.ifrc.org/sites/default/files/2021-06/NCD-care-humanitarian-settings-civil-society.pdf.

51. Muhammad H. Zaman, "The Quest for Ethical Solutions for the Global Refugee Crisis," Boston University, University Lecture, October 23, 2019, https://www.youtube.com/watch?v=vzgL6CRnyxs.

52. Nabil A. Nimer, "A Review on Emerging and Reemerging of Infectious Diseases in Jordan: The Aftermath of the Syrian Crises," *Canadian Journal of Infectious Diseases and Medical Microbiology*, May 24, 2018.

53. Lee W. Riley, Albert I. Ko, Alon Unger, and Mitermayer G. Reis, "Slum Health: Diseases of Neglected Populations," *BMC International Health and Human Rights* 7, no. 1 (2007): 1–6.

54. Naser Morina, Aemal Akhtar, Jürgen Barth, and Ulrich Schnyder, "Psychiatric Disorders in Refugees and Internally Displaced Persons after Forced Displacement: A Systematic Review," *Frontiers in Psychiatry* 9 (2018): 433.

55. Patrick Vinck, Phuong N. Pham, and Albert Ali Salah, "'Do No Harm' in the Age of Big Data: Data, Ethics, and the Refugees," in *Guide to Mobile Data Analytics in Refugee Scenarios*, ed. Albert Ali Salah, Alex Pentland, Bruno Lepri, and Emmanuel Letouzé (Springer Cham, 2019), 87–99.

56. Pia Vogler, "Into the Jungle of Bureaucracy: Negotiating Access to Camps at the Thai-Burma Border," *Refugee Survey Quarterly* 26, no. 3 (2007): 51–60.

57. "The World's Stateless," Institute on Statelessness and Inclusion, 2014, https://files.institutesi.org/worldsstateless.pdf.

58. Sebastian Schee Genannt Halfmann, Nikolaos Evangelatos, Emmanuel Kweyu, Carina DeVilliers, Kirsten Steinhausen, Alta Van der Merwe, and Angela Brand, "The Creation and Management of Innovations in Healthcare and ICT: The European and African Experience," *Public Health Genomics* 21, no. 5–6 (2018): 197–206.

59. A. Betts, L. Bloom, and N. Weaver, "Refugee Innovation: Humanitarian Innovation That Starts with Communities," Humanitarian Innovation Project, University of Oxford, 2015, https://www.rsc.ox.ac.uk/files/files-1/refugee-innovation-web-5-3mb.pdf.

60. See, for example, an ongoing effort at the American University of Beirut, the Humanitarian Engineering Initiative, https://www.aub.edu.lb/HEI/Pages/default.aspx.

61. IEEE hosts a Global Humanitarian Technology Conference (https://ieeeghtc.org), and there are routinely papers and presentations on refugee- and IDP-related issues.

62. One example of a hackathon for refugees is described in: Louise Brosset, "Learnings from Kenya on Post Hackathon Health Tech Project," Techfugees (website), June 24, 2021, https://techfugees.com/all_news/learnings-from-kenya-on-health-tech-projects/.

63. Vijay Sankaran, "This Is Why Hackathons Are Essentially Useless," Fast Company (website), November 15, 2019, https://www.fastcompany.com/90430416/this-is-why-hackathons-are-essentially-useless.

64. More information available at https://humanitariangrandchallenge.org.

65. Courtney Carson, "Trump Budget Proposes Steep Cuts to Research and Foreign Assistance That Will Threaten Global Health Research," Global

Health Technology Coalition, March 21, 2017, https://www.ghtcoalition
.org/blog/trump-budget-proposes-steep-cuts-to-research-and-foreign
-assistance-that-will-threaten-global-health-research.

66. Khorshed Alam and Sophia Imran, "The Digital Divide and Social
Inclusion among Refugee Migrants: A Case in Regional Australia,"
Information Technology & People 28, no. 2 (2015).

67. Ana Adronic, Marcin Lewandowski, and Evan Easton-Calabria, "Refugees and Digital Exclusion," Rethinking Refuge, University of Oxford
Refugee Studies Center, July 2021, https://www.rethinkingrefuge.org
/articles/refugees-and-digital-exclusion.

Chapter 7
Racism and Discrimination Impede Access to Health Care

1. Numerous cases have been reported, for an example; see John Montaño,
"'El Paseo de la Muerte' de la Primera Víctima Fatal de Coronavirus" ["'The
Walk of Death' of the First Coronavirus Victim"], *El Tiempo*, March 10,
2021, https://www.eltiempo.com/colombia/otras-ciudades/el-paseo-de-la
-muerte-que-sufrio-el-primer-fallecido-por-coronavirus-572273; and
"Migrante Presuntamente con COVID-19 Denuncia 'Paseo de la Muerte'"
["Migrant Allegedly Suffering from COVID-19 Denounces 'Walk of
Death'], Proyecto Migración Venezuela (website), July 8, 2020, https://
migravenezuela.com/web/articulo/denuncian-que-niegan-atencion-en-tres
-hospitales-a-venezolano-solicitante-de-refugio/2020.

2. Manuel Galindo-Arias, "Qué Hacer con los Médicos Extranjeros?"
["What to Do with Foreign Physicians?"], *Colombian Journal of Anesthe-
siology* 45, no. 2 (2017): 86–88.

3. "A Bengali Problem: Born in Pakistan but Stateless," Samaa Originals
(YouTube), December 18, 2021, https://www.youtube.com/watch?v
=2YGVggUyoPo.

4. Physician "brain drain" is quite common in Pakistan due to a variety of
economic and social factors. See, for example: Asfandyar Sheikh, Syed
Hassan Abbas Naqvi, Kainat Sheikh, Syed Hassan Shiraz Naqvi, and
Muhammad Yasin Bandukda, "Physician Migration at Its Roots: A Study
on the Factors Contributing towards a Career Choice Abroad among
Students at a Medical School in Pakistan," *Globalization and Health* 8,
no. 1 (2012): 1–11.

5. Joanne Lim, "Regenerating Informality in Machar Colony" (master's thesis, Politecnico di Milano, 2019), https://issuu.com/joannelimcy/docs/machar_colony_thesis_issuu_single.

6. "Karachi: 600 Patients Treated at Medical Camp, *Dawn*, May 26, 2002, https://www.dawn.com/news/37347/karachi-600-patients-treated-at-medical-camp.

7. Madiha Qureshi, "Education—A Beacon of Hope for Machar Colony's Impoverished Children," *Dawn*, July 14, 2015, https://www.dawn.com/news/1189964.

8. Zafirah Zein, "Hepatitis C Is Asia's Silent Emergency," *Kontinentalist*, July 28, 2021, https://kontinentalist.com/stories/hepatitis-c-kills-as-asia-struggles-to-get-treatment.

9. Mohammad Ayub Khan, *Diaries of Field Marshall Mohammad Ayub Khan, 1966–1972*, ed. Craig Baxter (Oxford University Press, 2008), 145.

10. Khan, *Diaries*, 145.

11. Mazhar Abbas, "Why Imran Idealises Ayub Era," *The News* (Pakistan), December 11, 2018, https://www.thenews.com.pk/print/404412-why-imran-idealises-ayub-era.

12. S. Akbar Zaidi, "A Reformer on Horseback," *Dawn*, September 2, 2017, https://www.dawn.com/news/1355171.

13. "A Bengali Problem: Born in Pakistan but Stateless," Samaa Originals (YouTube), December 18, 2021, https://www.youtube.com/watch?v=2YGVggUyoPo.

14. Shajeel Zaidi, "Is Pakistan Ready to Grant Citizenship to Its Afghan and Bengali Refugees?," *Express Tribune*, September 24, 2018, https://tribune.com.pk/article/72175/is-pakistan-ready-to-grant-citizenship-to-its-afghan-and-bengali-refugees.

15. Najam U. Din, *Internal Displacement in Pakistan: Contemporary Challenges*, Human Rights Commission of Pakistan, 2010, https://dev.humanitarianlibrary.org/sites/default/files/2014/02/22.pdf.

16. Philip Bump, "The Source of Black Poverty Isn't Black Culture, It's American Culture," *The Atlantic*, April 1, 2014, https://www.theatlantic.com/politics/archive/2014/04/the-source-of-black-poverty-isnt-black-culture-its-american-culture/359937/.

17. Carly Ching, Summiya Nizamuddin, Farah Rasheed, R. J. Seager, Felix Litvak, Faisal Sultan, and Muhammad Zaman, "Antimicrobial Resistance Trends from a Hospital and Diagnostic Facility in Lahore, Pakistan: A

Five-Year Retrospective Analysis (2014–2018)," *medRxiv* [pre-print] (2019): 19012617.

18. Sarah Kwon, "American Indians' Growing Presence in the Health Professions," *Health Affairs* 40, no. 2 (2021): 192–96.

19. Human Rights Watch, "Refugees, Asylum Seekers, Migrants, and Internally Displaced Persons," Report on the Fiftieth Anniversary of the 1951 Refugee Convention, 2002, https://www.hrw.org/legacy/wr2k2/refugees.html.

20. Zeina Chemali, F. L. Ezzeddine, B. Gelaye, M. L. Dossett, J. Salameh, M. Bizri, B. Dubale, and G. Fricchione, "Burnout among Healthcare Providers in the Complex Environment of the Middle East: A Systematic Review," *BMC Public Health* 19, no. 1 (2019): 1–21.

21. Bryony Lau, "Refugee-Run Organizations Deserve More Money," *Foreign Policy*, May 12, 2021, https://foreignpolicy.com/2021/05/12/refugee-run -organizations-deserve-more-money/.

22. Oliver Walton, "Humanitarian NGOs: Dealing with Authoritarian Regimes," *Bath Papers in International Development and Wellbeing*, Working Paper No. 42, Centre for Development Studies, 2015.

❙ Conclusion

1. Numerous pro-immigration groups make this argument; see, for example: National Immigration Forum, "Immigrants as Economic Contributors: Refugees Are a Fiscal Success Story for America," June 14, 2018, https:// immigrationforum.org/article/immigrants-as-economic-contributors -refugees-are-a-fiscal-success-story-for-america/.

Index